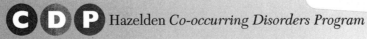
C D P Hazelden *Co-occurring Disorders Program*

*Integrated Services for Substance Use
and Mental Health Problems*

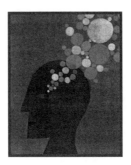

Clinical Administrator's Guidebook

Mark McGovern, Ph.D.
and other faculty from the Dartmouth Medical School

HAZELDEN®

Hazelden
Center City, Minnesota 55012
hazelden.org

ISBN: 978-1-59285-686-2

Editor's note

The names, details, and circumstances may have been changed to protect the privacy
of those mentioned in this publication.

This publication is not intended as a substitute for the advice of health care
professionals.

Alcoholics Anonymous and AA are registered trademarks of Alcoholics Anonymous
World Services, Inc.

The terms *mental health disorder, mental health problem,* and *psychiatric disorder*
are all used interchangeably throughout the Co-occurring Disorders Program. These
three terms refer to a non-severe diagnosis. The selection of terms used in each
component of the program may reflect the preference of the individual author.

Cover design by David Spohn
Interior design by Kinne Design
Typesetting by Kinne Design and Madeline Berglund

▼

ABOUT THE AUTHORS

Mark McGovern

Mark McGovern, Ph.D., is an associate professor of Psychiatry and of Community and Family Medicine at Dartmouth Medical School. Dr. McGovern specializes in the treatment of co-occurring substance use and psychiatric disorders and has studied and is published widely in the area of addiction treatment services research. In July 2004, he received a career development award from the National Institute on Drug Abuse. The overarching goal of this award involves developing, testing, and transferring evidence-based treatments to community settings for persons with co-occurring substance use and psychiatric disorders. Dr. McGovern recently received a grant from the Robert Wood Johnson Foundation to form and foster a multistate collaborative among addiction and mental health systems and treatment providers who are striving to improve the chances of recovery for their patients with co-occurring disorders.

Robert E. Drake

Robert E. Drake, M.D., Ph.D., is the Andrew Thomson professor of Psychiatry and of Community and Family Medicine at Dartmouth Medical School and the director of the Dartmouth Psychiatric Research Center. He has been at Dartmouth since 1985 and is currently vice chair and director of research in the Department of Psychiatry. He works as a community mental health doctor and researcher. His research focuses on co-occurring disorders, vocational rehabilitation, health services research, and evidence-based practices. He directs four national studies of quality improvement, and he has written fifteen books and more than four hundred papers about co-occurring disorders, vocational rehabilitation, mental health services, evidence-based practices, and shared decision making.

Matthew R. Merrens

Matthew R. Merrens, Ph.D., is codirector of the Dartmouth Evidence-Based Practices Center and a visiting professor of Psychiatry at Dartmouth Medical School. He received his Ph.D. in clinical psychology at the University of Montana and was formerly on the faculty and the chair of the Psychology Department at the State University of New York at Plattsburgh. He has extensive experience in clinical psychology and community mental health and has authored and edited textbooks on the psychology of personality, introductory psychology, the psychology of development, and social psychology. He recently published a book on evidence-based mental health practices. He is the director of the Dartmouth Summer Institute in Evidence-Based Psychiatry and Mental Health.

Kim T. Mueser

Kim T. Mueser, Ph.D., is a clinical psychologist and a professor of Psychiatry and of Community and Family Medicine at the Dartmouth Medical School in Hanover, New Hampshire. He received his Ph.D. in clinical psychology from the University of Illinois at Chicago in 1984 and was on the faculty of the Psychiatry Department at the Drexel University College of Medicine in Philadelphia until 1994. In 1994, he moved to Dartmouth Medical School and joined the Dartmouth Psychiatric Research Center. Dr. Mueser's clinical and research interests include integrated treatment for co-occurring psychiatric and substance use disorders, rehabilitation for persons with severe mental illnesses, and the treatment of post-traumatic stress disorder. He has published several hundred journal articles and has coauthored ten books.

Mary F. Brunette

Mary F. Brunette, M.D., is an associate professor of Psychiatry at Dartmouth Medical School. She has been working in the field of treatment for patients with co-occurring disorders for fifteen years. She conducts research on services and medications for people with co-occurring substance use and serious mental illness. She is a clinician who provides treatment for patients with co-occurring disorders. She also is medical director of the Bureau of Behavioral Health in the New Hampshire Department of Health and Human Services. She has published more than fifty articles and book chapters, many related to medication treatment for people with co-occurring disorders. She speaks nationally on this topic.

• • •

Integrated Services for Substance Use and Mental Health Problems

PROGRAM COMPONENTS

The Co-occurring Disorders Program is made up of a guidebook, five curricula, and a DVD. These components can stand alone, but when used together they provide a comprehensive, evidence-based program for the treatment of persons with co-occurring substance use and psychiatric disorders.

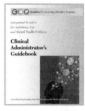 ← *Clinical Administrator's Guidebook*
Includes a guidebook and a CD-ROM.

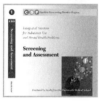 ← **Curriculum** ❶ *Screening and Assessment*
Includes a three-ring binder, a clinician's guide, and a CD-ROM.

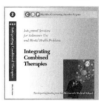 ← **Curriculum** ❷ *Integrating Combined Therapies*
Includes a three-ring binder, a clinician's guide, and a CD-ROM.

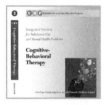 ← **Curriculum** ❸ *Cognitive-Behavioral Therapy*
Includes a three-ring binder, a clinician's guide, and a CD-ROM.

 ← **Curriculum** ❹ *Medication Management*
Includes a three-ring binder and a CD-ROM.

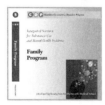 ← **Curriculum** ❺ *Family Program*
Includes a three-ring binder, a clinician's guide, and a CD-ROM.

 ← *A Guide for Living with Co-occurring Disorders: Help and Hope for Clients and Their Families*
Ninety-minute DVD.

▼

CONTENTS

▼

ACKNOWLEDGMENTS

The authors would like to express their gratitude to the many patients and programs who provided information about their treatment services. Without their candor and willingness the knowledge used to compile this guidebook would not be possible. Many patients, providers, treatment systems administrators, researchers, and colleagues have helped develop the Dual Diagnosis Capability in Addiction Treatment (DDCAT) Index. Critical to this effort include members of the multistate DDCAT Collaborative, including Julienne Giard, Rhonda Kincaid, Sabrina Trocchi, Kenneth Marcus, and Thomas A. Kirk Jr. from Connecticut; Jessica Brown, Joseph Comaty, and Tanya McGee from Louisiana; Ron Claus and Heather Gotham from Missouri; Joseph Harding, Lindy Keller, and James Shanelaris from New Hampshire; Cynthia Godin and Pamela Adelmen from Minnesota; John Viernes and David Garner from Indiana; Randi Tolliver, Phillip Welches, and Trina Diedrich from Illinois; Laurel Mangrum and Michelle Steinley-Bumgarner from Texas; and Paul Dragon and Kathy Browne from Vermont.

Special thanks should also be extended to John Challis and JoAnn Sacks at SAMHSA's Co-Occurring Center for Excellence (COCE). We are also grateful to our colleagues at the Dartmouth Psychiatric Research Center: Chantal Lambert Harris, Karen Becker, Gregory McHugo, William Torrey, and Haiyi Xie. Erica Ligeski provided steadfast and unfailing editorial support throughout the assembly and writing of this curriculum.

. . .

▼

PROGRAM OVERVIEW

Welcome to the **Co-occurring Disorders Program: Integrated Services for Substance Use and Mental Health Problems** developed by faculty from the Dartmouth Psychiatric Research Center, the Department of Psychiatry, and the Department of Community and Family Medicine, Dartmouth Medical School. This program focuses on integrated treatment of persons with concurrent substance use and non-severe mental health disorders, such as mood and anxiety disorders and less severe forms of bipolar disorder. This integrated treatment approach helps people recover by offering both mental health and substance use services at the same time and in one setting, or by the same providers.

The Co-occurring Disorders Program is made up of five curricula and two additional components that utilize print, DVD, and Web resources to serve the needs of all the primary stakeholders who treat and are affected by co-occurring disorders. Supervisors, clinicians, and health service workers will find educational materials to guide them in screening, assessing, and treating patients with co-occurring disorders. Worksheets, handouts, and video information are included for patients and their families. The program format is flexible enough to offer a standardized yet customizable treatment experience designed to give patients the maximum knowledge, structure, and support needed to allow them to achieve abstinence from drugs and initiate a long-term program of mental health recovery. Family members, along with patients, are encouraged and guided in the *Family Program* curriculum, which includes handouts and worksheets for educational purposes, as well as an instructional DVD that offers family members what they need to participate in the recovery of their loved ones.

***

Note: For the sake of convenience, the word "clinician" refers to any practitioner—counselors, supervisors, therapists, psychologists, facilitators, medical and mental health personnel, administrators, agency directors, and doctors—using these guides and curricula as part of the Co-occurring Disorders Program with patients and family members.

How Will the Co-occurring Disorders Program Help My Organization?

The goal of the Co-occurring Disorders Program is to help addiction treatment programs implement effective services for persons with non-severe mental health disorders that co-occur with a substance use disorder. However, the program can be used to treat these patients in mental health settings as well. Most addiction treatment providers recognize that patients with non-severe mental health disorders are already under their care. The program offers information and tools that will help you develop program policy, practice, and workforce resources in order to deliver the best care possible (in any setting) to all patients with co-occurring disorders.

What Is Included in the Co-occurring Disorders Program?

The Co-occurring Disorders Program includes a guidebook, five curricula, and a DVD that offer everything needed to create an integrated treatment program using the most current, evidence-based tools available.

The components of the Co-occurring Disorders Program are

▶ *Clinical Administrator's Guidebook*

This *Clinical Administrator's Guidebook* contains complete instructions for implementing the Co-occurring Disorders Program. The guidebook is for a mental health or addiction treatment organization's director, board of directors, CEO, CFO, and other key agency leaders. This guidebook offers all the tools a clinical administrator needs to assess the seven key areas of organizational effectiveness, including the policy, practice, and workforce benchmarks needed to deliver the best possible services to persons with co-occurring disorders. Chapters 4–13 serve as a valuable organizational assessment guide that outlines the steps needed to assess and improve services offered to patients with co-occurring disorders. Links to resources about co-occurring disorders, a sample charter agreement and Dual Diagnosis Capability in Addiction Treatment (DDCAT) Index implementation plan, and other materials are included on the accompanying CD-ROM.

▶ **Curriculum ❶** *Screening and Assessment*

Screening and Assessment is a must-use tool that helps clinicians evaluate patients with an effective, protocol-driven method so that appropriate treatment options can be addressed with regard to each patient's symptoms, disorder, and motivation to change. Included are specific measures for screening, assessment, differential diagnostics, and stage of motivation to address and treat both addiction and psychiatric problems in patients. *Screening and Assessment* comes with a bound clinician's guide and a CD-ROM with reproducible forms for clinicians packaged in a three-ring binder.

▶ **Curriculum ❷** *Integrating Combined Therapies*

Integrating Combined Therapies utilizes a combination of motivational enhancement therapy (MET), cognitive-behavioral therapy (CBT), and Twelve Step facilitation (TSF). Each of these therapy approaches has been proven successful when used in community addiction treatment programs. There is a growing consensus that these practices are effective if delivered singularly to patients, but are even more effective if rationally combined based on stage of motivation, problem pattern and severity, and patient preference. Each of these evidence-based practices is described here with appropriate modifications for persons with co-occurring disorders. At the time of this writing, these practices have not been adapted specifically for use in persons with co-occurring disorders, but readily lend themselves to this use with very simple augmentation. This curriculum will enable a clinician to successfully deliver these evidence-based therapies to patients with co-occurring disorders, which results in greater positive outcomes for patients. *Integrating Combined Therapies* comes with a bound clinician's guide and a CD-ROM with reproducible patient handouts packaged in a three-ring binder.

▶ **Curriculum ❸** *Cognitive-Behavioral Therapy*

Cognitive-Behavioral Therapy utilizes cognitive-behavioral therapy (CBT) principles to address the most common psychiatric problems in addiction treatment settings: mood and anxiety disorders and bipolar disorder. CBT is an evidence-based practice for treating substance use disorders and most psychiatric disorders. Research shows that CBT is useful for treating non-severe co-occurring psychiatric disorders in an addiction treatment setting. Psychosocial treatments, particularly CBT, are equally, if not more, effective for the psychiatric disorders that most commonly occur with substance use disorders. Research with CBT for persons with co-occurring disorders has been highly specialized by the specific co-occurring disorder. Providers had no one manual or practice, until now, to implement in real-world settings where patients have a variety of these disorders. Drawing from multiple manuals is burdensome for practitioners.

Cognitive-Behavioral Therapy includes a bound clinician's guide and a CD-ROM with reproducible patient handouts packaged in a three-ring binder.

▶ **Curriculum ❹** *Medication Management*

Medication Management is a valuable resource for medical directors and clinicians. It contains vital, current information about the complex issues of medication management, including medication compliance and other psychological concerns of the patient. Issues of differential diagnosis, timing, indications, monitoring, dosage, tolerance and withdrawal, and other issues are considered in this curriculum. Current evidence and consensus-based practices are provided to enable providers to make clinical decisions about medications and their prescription. While many people in peer recovery support groups take psychotropic medication, stigma can still cause some to hide their medication use from others. These issues, and information about the benefits and risks of medications, are also addressed for the patient. *Medication Management* comes with a CD-ROM and reproducible handouts packaged in a three-ring binder. It offers up-to-date, objective information for health care providers who prescribe medication or for clinicians who care for patients with co-occurring disorders who are using medications.

▶ **Curriculum ❺** *Family Program*

This curriculum helps clinicians involve patients with co-occurring disorders and their family members in an integrated treatment approach. First, family members, including the patient, meet to learn about the patient's specific psychiatric disorder and how it interacts with the substance use disorder. Then, the family joins other families in a twelve-week program of education on such topics as managing cravings, effective communication, using medications, and preventing relapses. The *Family Program* curriculum includes a clinician's guide and a CD-ROM with reproducible patient handouts packaged in a three-ring binder. In addition, a 90-minute DVD, *A Guide for Living with Co-occurring Disorders: Help and Hope for Clients and Their Families,* provides hope and healing for patients with co-occurring disorders and their family members.

▶ *A Guide for Living with Co-occurring Disorders: Help and Hope for Clients and Their Families*

This 90-minute DVD educates patients and families on the treatment of co-occurring disorders. It provides an educational overview of co-occurring disorders, shows interviews with people who have them, and discusses ways that patients can participate in treatment to better manage their recovery from both disorders. Included are dramatic vignettes as well as professional narration to show a comprehensive look at all the issues of recovery. Clinicians can use this DVD when implementing any of the five curricula of the Co-occurring Disorders Program.

An additional service available is

▶ *Training*

Implementation training developed by Hazelden with faculty of Dartmouth Psychiatric Research Center to help addiction treatment and mental health centers develop greater capacity, skills, and processes to treat non-severe mental health patients with substance use disorders is available. Dual Diagnosis Capability in Addiction Treatment (DDCAT) Index assessment training is also available from the faculty of Dartmouth Psychiatric Research Center and designated consultants from across the United States to help addiction treatment and mental health centers develop greater capacity, skills, and processes to treat non-severe mental health patients with substance use disorders.

Who Are the Authors of the Co-occurring Disorders Program?

The Co-occurring Disorders Program was developed and authored by faculty (listed below) from the Dartmouth Psychiatric Research Center, the Department of Psychiatry, and the Community and Family Medicine Department, Dartmouth Medical School at Dartmouth College. These faculty members are leaders in the field of co-occurring disorders in research, clinical experience, and expertise in addressing the complex issues in treating substance use and mental health disorders. Read the "About the Authors" section on pages iii and iv for a comprehensive description of each author's credentials and experience.

The Co-occurring Disorders Program authors are

- Mark McGovern, Ph.D., associate professor of Psychiatry and of Community and Family Medicine

- Robert E. Drake, M.D., Ph.D., professor of Psychiatry and of Community and Family Medicine

- Matthew R. Merrens, Ph.D., visiting professor of Psychiatry and codirector of the Dartmouth Evidence-Based Practices Center

- Kim T. Mueser, Ph.D., professor of Psychiatry and of Community and Family Medicine

- Mary F. Brunette, M.D., associate professor of Psychiatry

What Are the Goals of the Co-occurring Disorders Program?

The Co-occurring Disorders Program is consistent with the goal of the Dartmouth Psychiatric Research Center: To improve the lives of individuals and families affected by co-occurring disorders by creating and promoting evidence-based practices that increase the chances for recovery.

The primary goal of the Co-occurring Disorders Program is to offer current information and proven tools to effectively treat non-severe co-occurring disorders. The program is taken directly from research and best practices in the field.

This program

- helps program directors assess and expand the capabilities of their current organization

- offers clinicians an easy-to-use treatment program with tools that offer clients and their families the services and support needed

- integrates the most current best practices and therapies in the field, such as motivational enhancement therapy, cognitive-behavioral therapy, and Twelve Step facilitation

Is the Co-occurring Disorders Program Evidence-Based?

The Co-occurring Disorders Program combines best practices in substance use and mental health therapies into a comprehensive treatment program for patients with co-occurring disorders. The interventions in this program are primarily drawn from evidence-based therapies, such as cognitive-behavioral therapy, motivational interviewing, and Twelve Step facilitation.

The information provided in this *Clinical Administrator's Guidebook* of the Co-occurring Disorders Program is based on findings, observations, and studies of more than two hundred addiction treatment programs using the Dual Diagnosis Capability in Addiction Treatment (DDCAT) Index. The DDCAT was developed as a benchmark measure to assess an addiction treatment program's capacity to provide evidence-based treatment services to persons with co-occurring disorders. The benchmarks are based on expert consensus and evidence-based services for persons with co-occurring disorders. Drawing upon the numerous randomized controlled trials testing the Integrated Dual Disorder Treatment (IDDT) model, as well as the rapidly accumulating evidence base for practices with co-occurring substance use and non-severe mental health disorders, the Co-occurring Disorders

Program represents the state-of-the-science in treatment approaches for persons in addiction treatment settings. Since the evidence base for co-occurring disorders in addiction treatment exists on a continuum, each component of this series will describe the scientific status of the various treatment approaches, from investigative to promising to established practices. In some components—for example, the *Family Program*—careful adaptations of evidence-based approaches are made in order to be relevant for patients with non-severe psychiatric disorders in addiction treatment programs.

Who Can Use the Co-occurring Disorders Program?

The components of the Co-occurring Disorders Program are designed to be used by agency directors, administrators, supervisors, and clinicians. The program is designed for use with adult patients, as well as their family members, who are participating in a residential or outpatient treatment and/or mental health program for substance use and non-severe mental health disorders. These materials have been developed within the context of addiction treatment programs, but are equally useful when applied in a mental health program that would like to offer integrated treatment for co-occurring disorders.

Hard copies of handouts for patients (or forms for clinicians) are included in the three-ring binder of each curriculum. Reproducible copies of these handouts or forms are also available on the CD-ROM included with each curriculum. The treatment curricula of the Co-occurring Disorders Program (curricula ❷, ❸, and ❺) are suitable for individual or group therapy. Family members, friends, and other loved ones of patients are encouraged to participate in this program. Research shows that when family members are involved in the program, recovery for the patient is more likely.

How Is the Co-occurring Disorders Program Different from Other Programs?

The Co-occurring Disorders Program is specifically designed as an effective treatment program for patients with non-severe mental health disorders that co-occur with substance use disorders. The interventions in this program are evidence-based and primarily drawn from current research and practice in motivational interviewing, cognitive-behavioral therapy, and Twelve Step facilitation. This program is a comprehensive guide for clinicians, but also includes all the support tools necessary to implement an integrated treatment program to fulfill the needs of patients, family members, team members, and other stakeholders. In addition to four separate bound clinician's guides, these support tools include this *Clinical Administrator's Guidebook* (a program assessment guide), *Medication Management* for clinicians and medical directors, and *A Guide for Living with Co-occurring Disorders* (a 90-minute DVD for clinicians, patients, and family members).

Aside from Integrated Dual Disorder Treatment (IDDT), which is designed for persons with co-occurring disorders with severe mental illness (SMI), no other comprehensive manualized program exists for people with mental health disorders that co-occur with substance use disorders. The Co-occurring Disorders Program is based on the most current, comprehensive, evidence-based practices presently available.

How Are the Tools in the Co-occurring Disorders Program Different from the Integrated Dual Disorder Treatment (IDDT) Program?

The IDDT was developed and standardized for use primarily in mental health settings with persons with severe mental illness. The IDDT was not developed for and does not fit in most addiction treatment settings. The Co-occurring Disorders Program was created for use in addiction treatment settings for use with persons with non-severe psychiatric disorders who also suffer from any level (from low to severe) of substance use disorder. Non-severe mental health problems include depression and dysthymic disorders, anxiety disorders including post-traumatic stress disorder (PTSD) and social phobia, and bipolar disorders. For more severe mental illnesses, such as schizophrenia, schizoaffective disorder, severe major depression, and bipolar disorders, IDDT would be the model of choice. People using IDDT may choose to use the Co-occurring Disorders Program to expand their organization's capabilities to offer integrated treatment for people with non-severe psychiatric disorders.

Is the Co-occurring Disorders Program Compatible with Twelve Step Recovery?

For the program to be consistent with principles set forth in Alcoholics Anonymous (AA), Narcotics Anonymous (NA), and other recovery fellowships, the clinician should advocate and support the idea that the patient's best interest is for *abstinence* from *all* mood-altering substances, including alcohol, drugs, and any pharmaceuticals that the patient may be taking *without* a prescription. Patients are also encouraged to attend other peer recovery support groups, such as Dual Recovery Anonymous (DRA) or Double Trouble in Recovery (DTR). It is recommended that patients in this program purchase or be allowed to borrow copies of AA or NA publications. Furthermore, Twelve Step facilitation is covered in curriculum ❷ *Integrating Combined Therapies* as one of the three recommended evidence-based addiction treatment models.

What Special Issues Might Arise When Dealing with Different Cultural Groups?

The use of the Co-occurring Disorders Program interventions is not limited to certain races, ethnicities, or cultures. The educational information and inspirational stories included in the clinician's guides and in the program DVD depict and honor individual and cultural diversity.

This aspect of the Co-occurring Disorders Program makes it very appealing to people in many cultures. The delivery of information can be tailored to a particular population to make it as culturally specific as desired. The use of illustrations that depict diversity helps make the material more acceptable by a wide range of cultures and makes the information more easily understood by patients whose drug use and mental states have resulted in reduced cognitive abilities.

Is Training Necessary to Implement the Co-occurring Disorders Program?

Adherence and competence in implementation of the Co-occurring Disorders Program are associated with effective outcomes. It is recommended that you and/or your facility receive additional training and support from Hazelden Publishing and the Dartmouth Psychiatric Research Center to ensure quality implementation of the model. For information on training, customers may contact Hazelden Publishing at (800) 328-9000 or visit hazelden.org/cooccurring.

How Can I Start Using the Co-occurring Disorders Program?

Each of the components in the Co-occurring Disorders Program can stand alone, but when used together these components provide a comprehensive, evidence-based program for treatment of persons with co-occurring substance use and non-severe psychiatric disorders.

Distribute each component of the Co-occurring Disorders Program to the appropriate audience:

- *Clinical Administrator's Guidebook*
  This guidebook is appropriate for the program or agency director, board of directors, CEO, CFO, and other key agency leaders.

- **Curriculum ❶** *Screening and Assessment*

  This curriculum is appropriate for therapists, counselors, or clinicians.

- **Curriculum ❷** *Integrating Combined Therapies*

  This curriculum is appropriate for therapists, counselors, or clinicians.

- **Curriculum ❸** *Cognitive-Behavioral Therapy*

  This curriculum is appropriate for therapists, counselors, or clinicians.

- **Curriculum ❹** *Medication Management*

  The primary audience for this curriculum is medical directors, but it is also appropriate for therapists, counselors, or clinicians.

- **Curriculum ❺** *Family Program*

  This curriculum is appropriate for therapists, counselors, or clinicians.

- *A Guide for Living with Co-occurring Disorders: Help and Hope for Clients and Their Families*

  This 90-minute DVD is appropriate for therapists, counselors, or clinicians who will use the video to educate patients and their families.

Those seeking to make programmatic change should use all the components that make up the Co-occurring Disorders Program. Your attempts to enhance your program's services with these materials will be more successful if you form a program-steering committee, designate key individuals to implement and monitor the intended changes, and identify ways to sustain these changes. Some mechanisms to consider in sustaining organizational change include training, clinical supervision, and incorporating these changes into routine protocols (such as in your electronic medical record system).

Please follow the instructions provided at the beginning of each component. The sequence of the material is important to the creation of a treatment dynamic that moves the patient through a systematic recovery process.

• • •

CHAPTER 1

Introduction to the *Clinical Administrator's Guidebook*

The *Clinical Administrator's Guidebook* is the overall program guide to policy, practice, and the workforce skills necessary to deliver the best possible services to persons with co-occurring disorders. You may choose to use this guide to assess and make positive changes in seven key organizational areas that affect program policy, practice, and staffing.

What Is Included on the *Clinical Administrator's Guidebook* CD-ROM?

This *Clinical Administrator's Guidebook* includes a CD-ROM that contains journal articles, abstracts, and references to the relevant research conducted with co-occurring disorders. These treatment materials have evolved from the application of concepts, described in theoretical and applied research efforts, to the needs of patients with co-occurring disorders who are attempting to recover from drug and alcohol problems and, at the same time, to address their mental health disorders.

The CD-ROM also includes information about the Dual Diagnosis Capability in Addiction Treatment (DDCAT) Index, a set of objective policy, practice, and workforce benchmarks to assess your program's capacity to serve persons with co-occurring disorders.

The DDCAT can be used to evaluate your current program by asking questions that fall into seven key dimensions.

▶ **Dimension 1: Program Structure**

Do your overall program structure and policies help or inhibit providing services for individuals with co-occurring disorders?

▶ **Dimension 2: Program Milieu**

What is the "culture" of your program? Are the staff and physical environment welcoming and receptive to individuals with co-occurring disorders?

▶ **Dimensions 3 and 4: Clinical Process**

How do your clinical assessment and treatment procedures and protocols rate in relation to co-occurring disorder assessment and treatment?

▶ **Dimension 5: Continuity of Care**

How does your program handle continuing care and monitoring for individuals with co-occurring disorders?

▶ **Dimension 6: Staffing**

Do any staff members have expertise to assess and treat individuals with co-occurring disorders? What are the clinical supervision patterns of your program and hiring practices in regard to expertise in co-occurring disorders?

▶ **Dimension 7: Training**

Are staff adequately trained and supported for the assessment and treatment of individuals with co-occurring disorders?

How Can I Use the DDCAT Index?

Whether your organization is an addiction treatment center or a mental health center, you may want to use the assessment tools found in chapters 4 to 10 of this *Clinical Administrator's Guidebook* to measure the ability of your existing program to offer integrated treatment services for co-occurring disorders. For addiction treatment centers, the DDCAT Index will allow you to objectively measure your program at baseline. As your co-occurring treatment program changes and evolves, use the DDCAT as a periodic assessment (yardstick) to evaluate your organization's progress over time.

A companion, or sister, to the DDCAT, the Dual Diagnosis Capability in Mental Health Treatment (DDCMHT), has been developed by Heather Gotham of the Mid-America Addiction Technology Transfer Center, Jessica Brown and Joseph Comaty of the Louisiana Department of Health and Human Services, and Mark McGovern. The DDCMHT can assess the DDCAT-related benchmarks in mental health settings. Information about the DDCMHT is available from the Dartmouth Psychiatric Research Center and the Mid-America Addiction Technology Transfer Center.

 Links to the DDCAT and DDCMHT are on the CD-ROM that accompanies this guidebook.

What Does My DDCAT Score Mean?

The information in chapters 4 to 10 of this guidebook, along with the DDCAT Index or the DDCMHT, will help you categorize your addiction or mental health treatment program into one of four primary categories: addiction-only services (AOS), dual diagnosis capable (DDC), dual diagnosis enhanced (DDE), or mental health–only services (MHOS). The first three categories are adopted from the *American Society of Addiction Medicine Patient Placement Criteria-2nd edition revised (ASAM PPC-2R),* published in 2001. The category of MHOS is an adaptation of the DDCAT category (derived from the *ASAM PPC-2R*) of AOS. It is the comparable category for mental health settings as assessed using the Dual Diagnosis Capability in Mental Health Treatment (DDCMHT) Index. For this guidebook, much as the category of AOS pertains to addiction treatment programs' co-occurring capability, MHOS pertains to mental health programs' co-occurring capability.

Addiction-Only Services (AOS)

These addiction treatment programs cannot accommodate patients with co-occurring mental health disorders that require ongoing treatment, no matter how stable or functional the patient.

Mental Health–Only Services (MHOS)

These psychiatric treatment programs cannot accommodate patients with co-occurring substance use disorders that require ongoing treatment, no matter how stable or functional the patient.

Dual Diagnosis Capable (DDC)

Addiction treatment programs at the DDC level have a primary focus on treating substance use disorders. These programs are also capable of treating patients who have relatively stable diagnostic or sub-diagnostic co-occurring mental health disorders related to an emotional, behavioral, or cognitive disorder.

Mental health treatment programs at the DDC level have a primary focus on treating psychiatric disorders. These programs are also capable of treating patients who have relatively stable diagnostic or sub-diagnostic co-occurring substance use disorders.

Dual Diagnosis Enhanced (DDE)

These addiction treatment programs are designed to treat patients who have unstable or disabling co-occurring mental health disorders in addition to a substance use disorder.

These mental health treatment programs are designed to treat patients who have unstable or disabling co-occurring substance use disorders in addition to a psychiatric disorder.

In DDE-level programs, both mental health and substance use disorders are treated at the same time and same place, or by the same providers.

Who Should Evaluate Your Treatment Program?

To avoid potential bias, it's recommended that a person outside of your organization perform the DDCAT evaluation. Studies have consistently shown that self-assessments of program capacity, including using the DDCAT, yield inflated ratings of capability. There are numerous professionals who have been trained in the DDCAT methodology and who are available to perform assessments. Nonetheless, most persons who use the DDCAT have not been formally trained and still find it simple and straightforward to use. You can determine your own approach to doing a program DDCAT assessment and consider all the pros and cons for each possibility.

The DDCAT Index and associated scoring manuals, along with a list of professionals trained to perform the DDCAT evaluation, are available from the Dartmouth Web site at www.dms.dartmouth.edu/prc/dual/atsr.

 Please see the CD-ROM included with this guidebook for more information about the DDCAT Index, including research and methodology, sample DDCAT profiles, and links to DDCAT workbooks and scoring tools.

How Do I Start Using the *Clinical Administrator's Guidebook?*

Before you begin the program assessment work found in chapters 4 to 10 of this guidebook, please read the next chapter, "Overview of Co-occurring Disorders," for a brief history of research findings and information on the evolution and effectiveness of treatment models.

• • •

CHAPTER 2

Overview of Co-occurring Disorders

As in any discipline, sound training and experience are often keys to success. Before implementing the Co-occurring Disorders Program, please read this overview of co-occurring disorders. Included are important definitions, a history of the evolution of treatment, and information about key areas and agencies that affect funding and research.

What Are Co-occurring Disorders?

Some people suffer from a psychiatric or mental health disorder (such as depression, an anxiety disorder, bipolar disorder, or a mood or adjustment disorder) along with substance use of alcohol or other drugs. Or, a person may have had a substance use disorder at one time in his or her life (e.g., alcohol use in college), but may currently suffer from only one disorder (e.g., major depression). This combination of health disorders is often referred to as a dual diagnosis, dual disorders, or co-occurring disorders. Co-occurring disorders are common in the general population and are even more prevalent among persons seeking treatment in medical, mental health, or addiction treatment settings.

What Is a Substance Use Disorder?

For the purpose of this text, the term "substance use disorders" refers to both substance abuse and substance dependence (as defined by the *Diagnostic and Statistical Manual of Mental Disorders, Fourth Edition, Text Revision [DSM-IV-TR]* published by the American Psychiatric Association) and encompasses the use of both alcohol and other psychoactive substances. Though some see this term as ambiguous, it is used in this text because the lay public, politicians, and many substance use treatment professionals commonly use "substance abuse" to describe any excessive use of any addictive substance. In reality, most people with substance abuse–level disorders are not in addiction treatment. In fact, to be eligible for most addiction treatment settings, a substance dependence–level diagnosis is required.

How Many People Suffer from Co-occurring Disorders?

Researchers estimate that about half of the people treated in mental health settings have had at least one substance use problem in their lifetime, if not within the past year. Approximately 25 percent to 33 percent of the people treated in mental health settings also suffer from past-year or current substance use problems. In addiction treatment settings, these estimates are similar if not higher. As many as 50 percent to 75 percent of people in addiction treatment centers also suffer from a current psychiatric disorder, with an even higher percentage of people having suffered from a psychiatric disorder at some point in their lives.

What Is the Difference between Severe and Non-severe Mental Health Disorders?

Co-occurring substance use disorders occur in people with severe and non-severe mental health disorders. Severe disorders include schizophrenia, bipolar disorder, schizoaffective disorder, and major depressive disorders. Non-severe mental health disorders include mood disorders, anxiety disorders, adjustment disorders, and personality disorders. Of course, severity can vary substantially within any diagnostic condition. For example, depression can be mild, moderate, or severe. PTSD can likewise be well-managed or debilitating. Severity, therefore, is more complex than any specific disorder. However, for the purpose of organizing research, treatments, and policy, these gross categories have been found to be pragmatic and useful, even though they do not capture the inherent complexity and variabililty of the severity construct (McGovern et al., 2007; McGovern & McLellan, 2008).

Does Having a Co-occurring Disorder Affect Treatment Outcomes for Either Disorder?

Research shows that persons with co-occurring disorders (treated in either mental health or addiction treatment settings) have less favorable outcomes than persons who suffer from only addiction or only a psychiatric disorder. This means that if an alcoholic who is clinically depressed is admitted to an addiction treatment center, it's likely that he or she will receive less adequate treatment for depression than the non-addicted person who seeks depression treatment from a mental health provider. On the other side of the coin, if a depressed alcoholic and an ordinary alcoholic both enter an addiction treatment center, it's likely that the ordinary alcoholic will have a better chance at recovery from alcoholism than the depressed alcoholic.

Not all people with co-occurring disorders report poor treatment outcomes, but most experts agree that having a co-occurring disorder is best viewed as a "risk factor" that can lead to a negative treatment experience. Examples of poor outcomes that have been identified through research include dropping out of treatment early, frequent transfer of the patient between clinicians within treatment settings, recidivism and return to treatment, no decline in substance use, no improvement of psychiatric symptoms, suicide, victimization, increased use of medical services (including hospitals and emergency services), legal problems including incarceration, work and school problems, and less satisfaction with treatment. These negative treatment outcomes have not been lost on policymakers, research scientists, treatment providers, or individuals and families who suffer with co-occurring disorders.

Why Is Research on Co-occurring Disorders Challenging?

Researchers have sought to increase our knowledge of the best possible treatments for co-occurring disorders. Because of the complexity and heterogeneity of this field, the research has been cumbersome and slow to progress. One research challenge is in simply defining the term "co-occurring disorder." For example, a co-occurring disorder may be the co-existence of a diagnosis of schizophrenia and cannabis use, or a diagnosis of alcohol dependence and dysthymia. Further, a person may have had one disorder at one time in his or her life (e.g., alcohol use in college), but not presently, and may suffer at the moment from only one disorder (e.g., major depression). Since experimental rigor is an essential element to research, the need to more precisely define the differences and similarities among co-occurring disorder types has often made the translation of findings to clinical practice exceedingly difficult.

Over the past ten years, both the National Institute on Drug Abuse (NIDA) and the National Institute on Alcohol Abuse and Alcoholism (NIAAA) have increased research support for scientists seeking to develop and test treatments for persons with co-occurring disorders in addiction treatment settings. These institutes each have a different focus with respect to substances used by patients. (NIAAA focuses on alcohol use disorders; NIDA focuses on drug use disorders.) With the requirement for diagnostic precision in defining research samples, nationally sponsored research has been highly specific in focus. For example, NIDA has funded studies of cocaine-dependent women with PTSD, but these studies have excluded women with PTSD who also have Axis II personality disorders. The NIAAA has funded studies of alcohol-dependent persons with social phobia, but these studies have excluded persons with other substance use or psychiatric disorders. Precise diagnostic

Duplicating this page is illegal. Do not copy this material without written permission from the publisher.

7

combinations and strict inclusion criteria such as these may be important for research (i.e., studies have internal validity) but lack the ability to be extrapolated to real-world settings where patients tend to suffer from a complex mixture of mental health problems and addiction to various substances (i.e., studies need more external or ecological validity).

Pragmatic direction from the field of clinical research, both with respect to studies of medications and psychosocial therapies, have also been difficult for addiction treatment settings to come by. Further, research findings on persons without severe mental illnesses, but who suffer from depression, anxiety, or other "less severe" or disabling conditions have also been slow to accumulate.

Meanwhile, persons with non-severe mental health disorders along with substance use disorders still need professional help. They still need services. Addiction treatment providers and health care professionals struggle with old models of care. They try to provide the best possible treatment so that their patients may have at least an average chance (even though historical research suggests they have a less-than-average chance) at recovery.

Why Is the Assessment and Diagnosis of Co-occurring Disorders Challenging?

Historically, health care professionals who have attempted to treat patients with co-occurring disorders have tried to declare one of the disorders as "primary" and the other as "secondary" based on the order of onset, or some judgment about causality. For instance, if childhood sexual trauma precipitated symptoms of post-traumatic stress disorder (PTSD) and if alcoholism appeared in adulthood, then the perception was that the PTSD must be the primary diagnosis. Patients were treated first for the primary disorder under the assumption that this treatment would naturally leverage change in the secondary disorder. Generally, with the exception of substance-induced disorders, no evidence for therapeutic efficacy exists for this "primary" or "secondary" approach to treatment.

To complicate diagnosis, a person may have co-occurring disorders even though the mental health disorder and the substance use disorder do not occur simultaneously. For example, a patient may have suffered from a childhood behavioral disorder such as oppositional defiant disorder and now may present with cocaine dependence. Unless this person meets the present criteria for another psychiatric disorder (Axis I or Axis II disorders), he or she may not be assessed as having co-occurring disorders.

Many patients suffer from both substance use and psychiatric disorders, which are chronic (versus transient or acute). Current research shows that a past or recent past diagnosis of a psychiatric or substance use disorder (in the presence of its counterpart) may be sufficient to warrant a co-occurring disorder diagnosis.

A patient may have co-occurring disorders, and yet he or she may not presently exhibit enough symptoms (at the traditional diagnostic threshold) to be diagnosed with both disorders. Using traditional assessments tools, this patient would likely be diagnosed with only one disorder and would not receive adequate treatment for both disorders. This example demonstrates that assessment and diagnosis are important skills for both addiction and mental health clinicians. Please refer to curriculum ❶ *Screening and Assessment* for instructions and tools to conduct patient assessments.

What Are the Different Types of Co-occurring Disorders?

The heterogeneity of persons with co-occurring disorders is vast. A man with schizophrenia and cannabis abuse has as much of a co-occurring disorder as a woman with alcohol dependence and social phobia. Yet the potential for differential stigma, access to treatment, lifetime course of the disorder, extent of disability, evidence-based treatments, and peer recovery support groups will be vastly different.

One way of describing this heterogeneity is the quadrant model (also known as the New York model) for dual disorders (see figure 1). This model was featured in SAMHSA's *Report to Congress on the Prevention and Treatment of Co-occurring Substance Abuse Disorders and Mental Disorders* (published in 2002), and many find it to be of value in simplistically categorizing co-occurring disorder types. Evidence suggests that persons in quadrant III are more likely to present to addiction treatment programs since they suffer from dependence-level disorders. In contrast, persons from quadrant II will likely present to a mental health provider. Persons in quadrant I may not present for any formal addiction or mental health care but instead are more likely found in general health care settings. Persons in quadrant IV often present in crises to emergency rooms, psychiatric hospitals, and detoxification programs. Persons in quadrant IV have had challenges connecting to outpatient services in either addiction or mental health systems. Evidence-based strategies are still being developed for this segment of persons with co-occurring disorders.

The Co-occurring Disorders Program has been specifically developed for persons with non-severe mental health disorders who have any level (from low to high) of substance use disorder.

FIGURE 1

Quadrant Model for Co-occurring Psychiatric and Substance Use Disorders

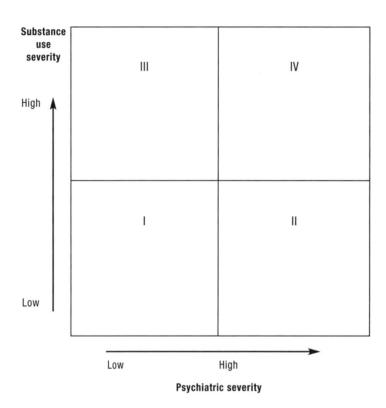

As figure 1 depicts, persons with co-occurring disorders may be categorized along two axes: psychiatric severity and substance use severity. A person with schizophrenia and cannabis abuse could arguably be placed in quadrant II. This person may be seen to suffer a problem with "high" psychiatric severity and relatively "low" substance severity. In contrast, a woman with social phobia and alcohol dependence could conceivably be placed in quadrant III because she may be seen to suffer from a less severe psychiatric disorder (social phobia versus schizophrenia) and a more severe substance use disorder (dependence versus abuse). Of course, many factors (disability, acuity) may also be associated with a diagnosis and severity. Therefore, many believe that this model is reductionistic and potentially obscuring of similarities and differences among persons with co-occurring disorders.

Meanwhile, professionals continue to use this model for its face validity and practicality. Recent research has validated the model for persons with co-occurring disorders in terms of prevalence and predicted treatment service utilization.

What Are the Basic Approaches to Treating Persons with Co-occurring Disorders?

Historically, the treatment of co-occurring disorders could be classified into four models, which are listed here in the order they have evolved. The first model (single model) offers the most basic approach to care, while the integrated model offers the most sophisticated.

The four models of care for co-occurring disorders are

1. Single model of care: The "primary" disease and treatment approach

2. Sequential model of care: Treating one disorder at a time

3. Parallel model of care: Concurrent treatment of both disorders (i.e., both disorders are treated at the same time but in different places)

4. Integrated model of care: Treating both disorders (i.e., both disorders are treated at the same time and at the same place, or by the same providers)

Despite the widespread use of the first three models, current research shows that an integrated approach to co-occurring disorder treatment results in the best possible patient outcomes.

1. Single Model of Care

Historically, the general assumption among mental health providers was that if an underlying mental health disorder was addressed, such as depression or anxiety, the patient would no longer need to use alcohol or other drugs to cope. Treatment focused on the underlying mental health disorder, with the belief that substance use would "drop off" or return to normal once the underlying disorder was resolved. This approach has been ineffective for substance use disorders and mental health problems.

This model of care is commonly termed the "self-medication" model. This model, at least from a mental health perspective, de-emphasizes the primary disease nature of addiction (substantiated in both human and animal studies), including all the biological and neurological changes associated with long-term substance use. The belief that addiction-related brain changes can be altered by addressing an underlying mental health condition alone is erroneous and without scientific foundation.

Duplicating this page is illegal. Do not copy this material without written permission from the publisher.

11

Conversely, addiction treatment professionals commonly witness profound if not miraculous changes in mood, anxiety, and self-esteem among patients who received only addiction treatment, including peer recovery group support. Addiction treatment providers often attribute treatment failure to those who drop out of services prematurely or who resist attending peer recovery support group meetings such as AA.

Patients who fare well under this treatment model are those who exhibit symptoms of a mental health disorder but do not have a "full-blown" disorder. For example, an alcoholic patient may suffer from symptoms of depression but not a depressive disorder. Recovery for this patient can be relatively straightforward, and the traditional "addiction-only services" approach for alcoholism is adequate. In contrast, an alcoholic who is clinically depressed may not experience relief from the symptoms of depression simply with abstinence from alcohol. This patient may require a more specific and targeted intervention for the equally severe co-occurring disorder of depression.

Although some patients will benefit from the primary disease and treatment approach, it is likely that those who have diagnosable disorders versus symptoms will require interventions directed at both conditions simultaneously.

2. Sequential Model of Care

The sequential treatment model suggests that a primary condition can only be dealt with once the underlying condition is treated so that it becomes less acute or at least less of an interference. For example, an addiction treatment professional may require a patient who is addicted to cocaine to be "stable psychiatrically" before addiction treatment can begin. The definition of stable may range from being "not actively suicidal" to being "capable of tolerating twelve hours of group therapy per day." Alternatively, in a mental health setting, a patient may be required to be "detoxed," or at least not high or intoxicated in order to be included in group therapy or to be seen by a clinician.

Sequential care does not facilitate the simultaneous utilization of both mental health and addiction treatment services. It may or may not conceptualize one of the disorders as primary, but does acknowledge that services may be necessary for both eventually, but not at the same time.

The sequential model essentially requires the patient to "hold off" on receiving services for one disorder while another disorder is the current focus of treatment. This "holding off" period may range from one week (as in, for example, a stay in an alcohol detoxification service) to six months (in residential treatment) to two years (as had been recommended for patients with PTSD who were in early recovery from substance use). In some cases, the sequential approach may be clinically reasonable (e.g., through withdrawal periods) and may help in confirming diagnostic impressions. Please refer to curriculum ❶ *Screening and Assessment* for instruction and tools to conduct patient assessments.

3. Parallel Model of Care

In this approach, specialty addiction treatment programs concurrently treat persons for addiction while they are in treatment at a mental health agency for a psychiatric disorder. This is known as parallel care or the concurrent model of care.

Parallel care happens in addiction treatment programs when addiction treatment services are provided while the patient is also being treated (pharmacologically or in individual psychotherapy) in a mental health setting for a psychiatric disorder. An addiction treatment program may recognize the need for mental health services—including, but not limited to, psychotropic medication—and may refer the patient for concurrent psychiatric evaluation and medication management. Likewise, a mental health professional may refer a psychiatric patient to an addiction treatment center for concurrent treatment for substance use.

Parallel services intend to provide care for both mental health and substance use disorders at the same time, but are typically offered in different settings and by different providers. Parallel care can be delivered in consultative, collaborative, or coordinated fashion (see the section entitled "How Do Treatment/Provider Relationships Vary within Models of Care?" beginning on page 14 for definitions of these terms). Parallel services often require the patient to navigate from provider to provider, or from program to program. Sometimes the communication between mental health and addiction providers is poor, and care is fragmented or duplicative or even conflictual. In other instances, parallel models are fairly well organized. Providers work in concert and as a team, even though they are from different programs in different locations. Services offered at the parallel level can approach integration if they are particularly well coordinated and the patient's experience can be relatively seamless.

4. Integrated Model of Care

Integrated treatment may take place at the individual clinician level, the program level, the agency level, or the system of care level.

An integrated clinician is one with developed expertise in both mental health and addictive disorders. Such professionals may have advanced certification in their discipline or mastery in specific treatment approaches.

Duplicating this page is illegal. Do not copy this material without written permission from the publisher.

13

Integration at the program level happens when members of a treatment team address both mental health and substance use disorders within a single treatment location, episode, record, and experience.

Integration at the agency level may share some, but not all, of the characteristics of programmatic integration, but more navigation by the patient and between clinicians is required. In this instance, an agency may provide both addiction and mental health services but in separate programs or departments. The patient may be asked to meet with two sets of providers, who may vary in clear lines of communication about the treatment plan or the patient's response to treatment.

Integration may also exist at the system level, such as within a geographical region, where clear guidelines and linkages are seamless and formalized. In this instance, two separate agencies may have a well-developed protocol for simultaneously managing patient care. Agencies may share as many as 25 percent of the same patients and have worked out ways to develop a common treatment plan and to monitor patient progress.

Integration requires the active collaboration of both addiction and mental health services providers in the development of a single treatment plan to address both disorders. It also requires the continuing formal interaction and cooperation of these providers in the ongoing reassessment and treatment of the patient.

How Do Treatment/Provider Relationships Vary within Models of Care?

Models of care may vary by the nature and type of relationship that exists between the addiction and mental health services professionals.

The following terms are used to describe these relationships:

1. Minimal coordination

2. Consultation

3. Collaboration

4. Integration

These terms represent the nature and quality of the relational contact and coordination between service providers. They do not refer to the program structure or location. "Minimal coordination" is the lowest benchmark while "integration" is the highest.

1. Minimal Coordination

A program could be functioning at the level of minimal coordination even though mental health and addiction treatment services are being provided by two people working at the same agency in the same building; whereas, another program could be at the integration level even if services are provided by two people working for different agencies in different programs. In other words, "co-location" guarantees nothing. The relationship may be integrated or minimal regardless of shared space.

Programs at the level of minimal coordination may acknowledge a co-occurring condition; however, there is no effort made to handle the condition. On the rare occasion that a referral is made, the follow-up is typically inadequate.

2. Consultation

Programs at the level of consultation may have informal and limited interactions with outside service providers. This may involve transferring medical/clinical information or giving updates on a patient's progress. The key to this level is that the program attempts to maintain a connection after the initial referral to ensure the referred person enters the recommended treatment service.

3. Collaboration

Programs at the level of collaboration formally and systematically involve multiple service providers in the sharing of responsibility for treating a person with co-occurring disorders. This includes regular and planned communication, sharing of progress reports, or memoranda of agreement. The key to this level is that all parties involved are aware of their responsibilities and expectations.

4. Integration

Programs at the level of integration involve members of a treatment team working together to cover both mental health and substance use disorders within a single treatment location, episode, record, and experience. Parallel models can approach integration contingent upon the degree of coordination. Some sequential models can also approach integration if the process of linkage is seamless from the clinical and patient perspective. This guidebook will describe how services can be delivered to support integration, even in parallel or sequential frameworks.

How Is the Treatment of Co-occurring Disorders Improving?

Historically, health care organizations have often failed to approach and treat psychiatric disorders and addiction as concurrent disorders requiring concurrent treatment. In fact, about 50 percent of persons with co-occurring disorders never receive concurrent treatment for both disorders. In cases where concurrent treatment is offered, 75 percent to 85 percent of the time those services are not offered

Duplicating this page is illegal. Do not copy this material without written permission from the publisher.

15

in an integrated manner. This probably leaves less than 15 percent of persons with co-occurring disorders receiving adequate treatment.

Over the past twenty years, increasing efforts have been underway to make positive changes in systems of care. These changes include how, what, and where treatment is delivered, as well as how these services are paid for by third parties such as Medicaid, Medicare, federal block grants, and private insurance companies. Parallel efforts have been occurring even more recently to address workforce issues. In the meantime, current research demonstrates that integrated treatment, which treats both disorders concurrently, offers the best possible outcomes for patients and patients' families. The Co-occurring Disorders Program offers a guidebook, five curricula, and a DVD that create a comprehensive program of evidence-based, integrated treatment for co-occurring disorders.

•   •   •

Introduction to Dual Diagnosis
Capability Program Assessment

CHAPTER **3**

Chapters 4 through 10 of this *Clinical Administrator's Guidebook* cover the policy, clinical practice, and workforce resources that organizations must evaluate when assessing their capability to serve persons with co-occurring disorders. This guidebook includes all the tools needed to evaluate, improve, and track your organization's capabilities.

As with the DDCAT treatment program assessment tool, the chapters in the *Clinical Administrator's Guidebook* are organized by seven dimensions that fall under one of three categories: policy, clinical practice, and workforce.

POLICY	CLINICAL PRACTICE	WORKFORCE
1. Program structure 2. Program milieu	3. Assessment 4. Treatment 5. Continuity of care	6. Staffing 7. Training

Chapters 4 through 10 offer specific instruction on how to evaluate your organization within each of the seven organizational dimensions and offer examples of why each dimension is important.

Before you proceed into the detailed analysis beginning in chapter 4, read this brief overview of the seven dimensions. This overview identifies the key people who affect each dimension. It also lists the key questions that staff should ask themselves to evaluate their organization's capabilities within each dimension.

POLICY

1. Program Structure

Who Are the Key People Who Establish a Program's Policy?

Key people include an agency director, board of directors, key agency administrative and clinical leadership, the CEO, the CFO, and sometimes—through a consumer advisory board or committee—former patients and patients' families.

What Are the Key Questions for Your Organization?

- What kind of agency do we have?

- What is our mission statement and what is involved in changing it?

- What are our present financial and licensing arrangements for mental health services, or for persons with mental health diagnoses?

- What kind of relationship do we have with the local mental health service providers who we refer patients to most frequently?

2. Program Milieu

Who Are the Key People Who Create the Physical or Social Environment in Which Treatment Occurs?

Key people include an agency director, board of directors, key agency administrative and clinical leadership, the CEO, the CFO, and patients and patients' families.

What Are the Key Questions for Your Organization?

- What kind of social and physical environment do we have?

- What does our environment, including the decor, posters, artwork, and brochures, say about our receptivity to persons with psychiatric problems?

- Is there a stigma to having a psychiatric problem?

- Do we welcome everyone?

- Are there patient and family education materials about co-occurring disorders that are available in the waiting areas and on the walls, or incorporated into group or individual sessions?

CLINICAL PRACTICE

3. Assessment

Who Are the Key People Who Affect Patient Assessment?

Key people include agency administrative and clinical leadership, clinical supervisors, and clinicians.

What Are the Key Questions for Your Organization?

- What is our current protocol to screen, assess, and diagnose psychiatric disorders?

- How do we make distinctions between symptoms, substance-induced disorders, or actual psychiatric disorders that may need treatment?

- Is our assessment protocol systematic or does it vary, depending on the particular clinician who performs the assessment?

- Do we have exclusion criteria based on psychiatric issues?

- Who reviews and enforces these criteria and what are his or her qualifications?

- Do we think about, talk about, or document patient motivation and preferences for treatments during our initial encounter?

4. Treatment

Who Are the Key People Who Affect Patient Treatment?

Key people include agency administrative and clinical leadership, clinical supervisors, and clinicians.

What Are the Key Questions for Your Organization?

- What do we do about our patients' psychiatric problems?

- What kind of access to medications do our patients have?

- Do we have therapy groups, educational sessions, or family sessions that discuss psychiatric issues?

- Do we consider the special challenges a person with co-occurring disorders may face when attending community peer recovery support group meetings?

- Do we think about, talk about, or document patient motivation and preferences for treatments and adapt what we offer them based on these considerations?

5. Continuity of Care

Who Are the Key People Who Affect Continuity of Care?
Key people include agency administrative and clinical leadership and clinicians.

What Are the Key Questions for Your Organization?

- What happens if a patient under our care is suicidal, homicidal, unable to care for herself or himself, unable to sit for a full day in our group program, unable to get out of bed, unable to talk in groups, and/or unable to stop thinking about troubling memories?

- Does our treatment with a patient have an endpoint?

- Do we encourage patients who have successful recovery to come back and share their stories with current patients?

- When we discharge or transfer patients do we consider psychiatric needs?

WORKFORCE

6. Staffing

Who Are the Key People Who Have Direct Contact with Patients?
Key people include agency administrative and clinical leadership, administrative support staff, clinical supervisors, clinicians, and peer recovery support persons. Also, personnel such as residential aides or other paraprofessionals may play an influential role.

What Are the Key Questions for Your Organization?

- Do our patients have ready access to medications that are evidence-based (i.e., FDA-approved) for psychiatric problems?

- What role does the person who prescribes this medicine play in our program?

- Do we have staff members who are capable and supported in assessing and offering treatment to persons with co-occurring psychiatric problems?

- What mechanisms do we have to supervise and review care for persons with psychiatric problems?

- How open are we to persons in recovery from co-occurring disorders being a part of our service delivery team?

7. Training

Who Are the Key People Who Have Patient Contact and How Are They Trained?
Key people include agency administrative and clinical leadership, administrative support staff, clinical supervisors, clinicians, and peer recovery support persons. Also, personnel such as residential aides or other paraprofessionals may play an influential role.

What Are the Key Questions for Your Organization?

- Are all agency personnel, patients, and families accepting and open about psychiatric problems?

- Do the majority of our clinical staff know which psychiatric disorders are most likely present in persons under their care, how to identify them, and what to do about them?

- How many clinical staff members are competent in delivering an evidence-based treatment to persons with co-occurring disorders?

- Do we keep track of the money and time we spend on training, and do we dedicate a portion of training to co-occurring disorders?

▼

In chapters 4 to 13 of this *Clinical Administrator's Guidebook,* you will find specific recommendations and practical tools to address each of the seven organizational dimensions that organizations must consider when developing or improving services for persons with co-occurring disorders.

Keep in mind the role of all key people who may be interested in or charged with implementing these best practices. Change can be challenging and takes time, but with strong leadership, patience, and a team united toward the same goal, you can be very successful in creating or expanding your organization's capabilities to offer integrated treatment for people with co-occurring disorders.

• • •

Policy:
Evaluating Your Program Structure

If you are seeking to create or improve integrated treatment for persons with co-occurring disorders, one of your first steps is to evaluate your program's policy, which includes the program structure that your organization operates within and the program milieu that communicates your program goals to the general community and to patients.

POLICY
1. Program structure
2. Program milieu

Chapter 4 will help you evaluate your current program structure. In chapter 5 you will complete your policy assessment by inspecting your program milieu.

Understanding Your Program Structure Barriers

When addiction treatment or mental health providers look critically at their organization, they may find that the three primary components of program structure—billing, financing, and licensure of services—are limiting or undermining efforts to provide integrated services for co-occurring disorders.

Financing of services is a significant issue that affects all organizations. When you evaluate your program structure, you will want to consider the types of services you can bill for and what diagnoses patients must have in order for invoices to be cleanly processed. Further, in the case of federal block grant dollars, each state may be required to distribute funds to public sector providers, either through the Center for Substance Abuse Treatment (United States Department of Health and Human Services, Center for Substance Abuse Treatment) or the Center for Mental Health Services (United States Department of Health and Human Services, Center for Mental Health Services) contracts. This means that a provider, depending on the state where the organization operates, may not be able to bill for mental health services within their agency, or they may not be able to bill for a unit of service for a person who is not "primarily" diagnosed with a substance use disorder.

Program licensure is another significant issue that affects all organizations. For example, some addiction treatment programs are only licensed to provide services to people with substance use disorders—not psychiatric disorders. If an

CLINICAL ADMINISTRATOR'S GUIDEBOOK

> **PROGRAM STRUCTURE BENCHMARKS**
>
> Program structure refers to four specific benchmarks:
>
> 1. Mission statement
> 2. Licensure and certifications
> 3. Relationships with outside professionals
> 4. Billing mechanisms

alcoholic with clinical depression presents at one of these treatment centers, then services can be delivered for the substance use disorder only. This means that the patient will not receive treatment for the co-occurring depression disorder. On the other hand, some mental health settings are not licensed to offer addiction treatment for people who have a psychiatric disorder along with a substance use disorder. These structures limit a program's ability to offer and bill for integrated treatment. These policies on billing and licensure are frequently driven at the state level, but other local or regional authorities such as counties, parishes, or municipalities may also determine them.

Many agencies have sought to overcome organizational structure challenges by obtaining licensure or certification for both addiction and mental health treatment. Other agencies have developed the capability to bill for mental health services à la carte or in unbundled formats, while still billing for program services (e.g., residential bed day or intensive outpatient unit of service) in the more traditional manner.

Third-party financiers, such as private health insurance companies, have developed slightly more flexible policies in this respect, although they often encourage sequential treatment by discouraging the simultaneous treatment of two conditions (addiction and psychiatric disorder).

For these reasons, it is critically important to understand what your organization's policies are in terms of licensure and billing parameters. It's important to stay aware of recent developments in your state and community to support integrated treatment, whether by more appropriate financing methods or certifications. This will allow you to base your treatment policies on present rather than historical information.

As more co-occurring treatment information is distributed and accepted—through clinical practice and research, and through the ongoing education of patients and families—policymakers and financiers of these services will be increasingly pressured to remove unnecessary barriers to integrated treatment.

In the sections that follow, the four program structure benchmarks are defined in detail and examples of programs that are operating at dual diagnosis capable (DDC) and dual diagnosis enhanced (DDE) levels are given. Suggestions for how a program could enhance its performance on each benchmark are also given.

Mission Statement

What is your agency's mission statement and does it recognize co-occurring disorders and the mandate to treat them? An organization's mission statement is a declaration of the overarching goals and values of the agency. It should define not only what the agency is, but also what the agency aspires to be. This declaration communicates your organization's identity and purpose to the community. Mission statements are often found in program brochures, promotional materials, employee manuals, or in frames on walls of offices or waiting areas.

Mission statements can and should be updated to reflect an organization's philosophy on treatment. This may involve a thoughtful process among agency leadership, a board of directors or advisors, frontline staff, patients, and members of the community. For example, if a program intentionally offers treatment for individuals with co-occurring disorders, the mission statement should reflect this. Many programs have had the same mission statement since their origins.

> *"We provide help and hope to persons and families suffering from alcoholism."*

This is a good mission statement. It is clear, and it is positive. But notice that this mission statement focuses on alcoholism, which leads people to wonder if treatment is offered for cocaine or other drug dependence.

Depending on the type of treatment your organization offers (see page 27 for a description of the various types of services), you may already use one of these five mission statements:

- Organizations that treat addiction only (AOS level) may say: "Organization X assists persons with alcohol and drug problems and helps them regain control over their lives."

Evaluate Your Mission Statement

When evaluating your organization's mission statement ask

- What does your mission statement say about the identity of your agency?

- Does your mission statement identify the type of treatment offered for people with co-occurring disorders? Is integrated treatment one of your program's primary objectives?

- Is your organization's identity reflected in the way counselors, clinicians, and patients intersect?

- How does your mission statement translate into actual practice?

- Organizations that treat mental health disorders only (MHOS level) may say: "Organization X assists persons with mental health disorders and helps them regain control over their lives."

- Organizations that treat addiction, but with the expectation and willingness to treat those with co-occurring disorders (DDC level) may say: "The mission of Organization X is to provide treatment to adults and adolescents with addictive disorders. Organization X ensures that all patients have access to behavioral health services."

- Organizations that treat mental health disorders, but with the expectation and willingness to treat those with co-occurring disorders (DDC level) may say: "The mission of Organization X is to provide treatment to adults and adolescents with mental health disorders. Organization X ensures that all patients have access to addiction treatment services."

- Organizations that treat persons with co-occurring disorders and have the capacity to offer integrated treatment for both mental health and substance use disorders (DDE level) may say: "Organization X is a private nonprofit organization dedicated to supporting the recovery of families and individuals who experience co-occurring mental health and substance use disorders."

Improve Your Mission Statement

Your mission statement is reflective of your program goals and philosophies. It communicates your identity. Changing the mission statement of your program does not necessarily mean that the activities or practices will change, but it does indicate that the program's leadership is moving in a new direction. Sometimes, changing the mission statement causes an enormous shift in outlook.

If you are seeking to expand your program to move from addiction-only services (AOS) or mental health–only services (MHOS) to dual diagnosis capable (DDC), then start by crafting a mission statement that communicates the fact that your program treats mental health and substance use disorders equally.

Licensure and Certifications

What are your program's licensure and certifications? Do they help or hinder attempts to provide services to persons with co-occurring disorders? To provide enhanced services to persons with co-occurring disorders, your organization must possess the appropriate licenses and certifications for treatment of both psychiatric disorders and substance use disorders. If your organization does not possess the required licenses and certifications, the types of services you can deliver will be restricted.

Addiction treatment organizations that are licensed and certified to treat only substance use are often faced with treating people who also have a psychiatric disorder. Research suggests that although these addiction treatment programs may intend to "deflect" patients with more acute (e.g., suicidality) or disabling

Program Definitions

Addiction-Only Services (AOS)

These addiction treatment programs cannot accommodate patients with co-occurring mental health disorders that require ongoing treatment, no matter how stable or functional the patient.

Mental Health–Only Services (MHOS)

These psychiatric treatment programs cannot accommodate patients with co-occurring substance use disorders that require ongoing treatment, no matter how stable or functional the patient.

Dual Diagnosis Capable (DDC)

Addiction treatment programs at the DDC level have a primary focus on treating substance use disorders. These programs are also capable of treating patients who have relatively stable diagnostic or sub-diagnostic co-occurring mental health disorders related to an emotional, behavioral, or cognitive disorder.

Mental health treatment programs at the DDC level have a primary focus on treating psychiatric disorders. These programs are also capable of treating patients who have relatively stable diagnostic or sub-diagnostic co-occurring substance use disorders.

Dual Diagnosis Enhanced (DDE)

These addiction treatment programs are designed to treat patients who have unstable or disabling co-occurring mental health disorders in addition to a substance use disorder.

These mental health treatment programs are designed to treat patients who have unstable or disabling co-occurring substance use disorders in addition to a psychiatric disorder.

(e.g., schizophrenia) psychiatric issues, a considerable proportion of patients will suffer non-severe mental health disorders (mood, anxiety, PTSD, or other problems) that complicate addiction treatment. Thoughtful programs are advocating for policy change to reflect this fact. Some addiction treatment programs have made conscious choices to provide mental health services—sometimes at a loss or break-even financial level—to give their patients the best shot at recovery.

Evaluate Your Licensure and Certifications
Make sure you understand the rules and regulations that your organization abides by. Programs seeking to enhance services will need to address the licensure and certification benchmark item at an administrative, bureaucratic, and policy level.

Improve Your Licensure and Certifications
Some treatment programs may be limited in what they can provide based solely upon licensure and certifications. Programs seeking to enhance their services must first verify if restrictions from state or regional policies actually exist. In some instances, the best way to provide integrated treatment for both mental health and substance use disorders is to gain joint mental health and addiction treatment licensure or hire licensed staff to bill for unbundled services.

Some programs may choose to "accept" their current structural barriers and instead focus on enhancing benchmarks in the other dimensions, such as program

---

Evaluate an Addiction or Mental Health Treatment Program

*In general, a program's **licensure or certifications** may fall into one of five categories.*

The program may
- restrict services to treat only individuals with substance use disorders.
- restrict services to treat only individuals with psychiatric disorders.
- offer services for individuals with co-occurring disorders, but identify the primary population, or patients, to be those with substance use disorders. (Often the staff and administrators of this type of organization believe they cannot provide treatment for mental health disorders.)
- offer services for individuals with co-occurring disorders, but identify the primary population, or patients, to be those with mental health disorders. (Often the staff and administrators of this type of organization believe they cannot provide treatment for substance use disorders.)
- offer services for individuals with co-occurring disorders by providing services for both mental health and substance-related disorders.

milieu, clinical process, continuity of care, staffing, or training. In addiction treatment centers this approach treats mental health problems as "complications" or "threats to recovery." The *American Society of Addiction Medicine Patient Placement Criteria-2nd edition revised (ASAM PPC-2R)* incorporates "emotional, behavioral, and cognitive complications" into the ASAM multidimensional model (dimension III). Using the ASAM Patient Placement Criteria more precisely has enabled some providers to provide psychiatric services (targeting dimension III) without changing licensure. However, addiction treatment programs that are already dual diagnosis capable and are looking to enhance their services may be able to acquire additional licensure or certification to provide mental health services. The same is true of mental health programs that may be able, through licensure or certification, to enhance their addiction treatment services.

For more information on ASAM Patient Placement Criteria, see page 30.

Relationships with Outside Professionals

In your program, what is the nature and quality of the relationship between addiction treatment and mental health services? When any program begins to provide enhanced services to people with co-occurring disorders, there is typically an increase in the amount of communication and shared responsibility between the program and outside providers who offer services for addiction treatment and psychiatric disorders.

Evaluate Your Relationships with Outside Professionals

The shared responsibilities and relationships between addiction treatment and mental health services providers fall into four different categories with "minimal coordination" as the lowest benchmark and "integration" as the highest. Take a look at your treatment program and determine which of the following categories best describes your relationships with outside professionals.

1. Minimal coordination—Addiction or mental health programs at this level may acknowledge a co-occurring condition; however, there is no effort made to link to outside agencies to handle the condition. On the rare occasion that a referral is made, the follow-up is typically inadequate. These programs are at the AOS or MHOS level.

2. Consultation—Addiction or mental health treatment programs at the consultation level may have informal and limited interactions with outside service providers. This may involve transferring medical/clinical information or giving updates on a patient's progress. The key to this level is that the

ASAM Patient Placement Criteria

1. Acute Intoxication and/or Withdrawal Potential
Risk associated with the patient's current level of acute intoxication; current signs of withdrawal; significant risk for severe symptoms or seizures upon withdrawal based on previous withdrawal history or current use patterns; ambulatory detoxification.

2. Biomedical Conditions and Complications
Current chronic medical conditions or physical illnesses (other than withdrawal) that may complicate treatment; need to address conditions prior to beginning treatment.

3. Emotional, Behavioral, or Cognitive Conditions and Complications
Current psychiatric disorders—behavioral, emotional, or cognitive—that may complicate treatment; chronic conditions; addictive disorders that require mental health treatment; ability to deal with activities of daily living.

4. Readiness to Change
Awareness of the need to change; level of commitment and readiness for change; likelihood to cooperate with treatment; recognition of the negative consequences of alcohol and/or drug use.

5. Relapse/Continued Use, Continued Problem Potential
Potential for relapse or continued use; ability of the patient to identify his or her relapse triggers; patient's coping skills.

6. Recovery Environment
Family members, significant others, and living, work, and school environments that may pose a threat to treatment or recovery; issues such as child care, housing, employment, or transportation that may pose a threat to treatment or recovery; availability of supportive friends or financial, educational, and vocational resources to assist in treatment or recovery.

For a link to the American Society of Addiction Medicine Web site, see the CD-ROM included with this guidebook.

program attempts to maintain a connection after the initial referral to ensure the referred person enters the recommended treatment service. These programs have almost reached the DDC level; they have exceeded minimal coordination but have not reached collaboration.

3. Collaboration—Programs reach the collaboration level when they formally and systematically involve multiple service providers in sharing responsibility for treating a person with a co-occurring disorder. This includes regular and planned communication, sharing of progress reports, or memoranda of agreement. The key to this level is that all parties involved are aware of their responsibilities and expectations. In advanced collaboration, the addiction and mental health professionals demonstrate some elements of integration. However, these elements of integration are not formal and are not defined within the program structure. These programs have reached the DDC level.

4. Integration—Programs are at the level of integration when members of a treatment team work together to cover both mental health and substance use disorders within a single treatment location, episode, record, and experience. A program's care is considered "integrated" rather than "collaborative" when the program has shared responsibility for the development and implementation of a treatment plan that addresses the co-occurring disorder. These programs have reached the DDE level.

An important aspect of these relationships is the degree to which they are formalized and systematic. Many AOS programs rely on local mental health providers to care for the medication, psychiatric emergency, psychiatric hospitalization, and sometimes the psychotherapeutic needs of their patients. MHOS programs rely on addiction treatment providers to provide specialized services for addiction such as detoxification, anti-addiction medications (such as buprenorphine), or even motivational enhancement, relapse prevention, or recovery groups.

DDC programs may provide more services than AOS and MHOS programs for addiction and mental health within the context of their location. DDE programs may provide even more addiction and mental health services than DDC programs that are also directed to a broader range of persons. For DDC programs to move to the DDE level, DDC programs should provide all services to patients "in house" to reduce the need to seek services from an outside provider.

Create a Charter Agreement

When some of an organization's co-occurring treatment services are provided off-site or by an external provider on-site, the nature of the relationships between the organization and these external providers should be considered. Sometimes these relationships are very informal and clinician-driven. For example, Amanda is a clinician that previously worked at the South Main Street Counseling Center (addiction program), but now works at St. Mary's Hospital (psychiatric program). Patients from South Main can see a doctor at St. Mary's Hospital because the clinicians at South Main can call Amanda and she can fast-track them into the psychiatric program. While this system can work, and is commonplace in many community settings, it is also the case that if Amanda were to leave her position (note the high rate of turnover in the addiction and mental health professions), this collaboration-level relationship would be in considerable jeopardy.

For this reason, this benchmark that measures relationships with outside professionals values relationships that are documented and systematic and maintained at a higher level. A "charter agreement" or "memorandum of understanding," along with regular meetings among key clinical leaders, are two examples of how to increase the systematization of these relationships. One hopes that these measures do not undermine the personal relationships frontline clinicians will develop; however, they afford an agency a measure of insurance against inevitable changes in personnel.

 A practical example of a charter agreement is included on the CD-ROM that accompanies this guidebook. This charter agreement can be customized for your use to systematize your relationship with providers of psychiatric or mental health services.

Improve Your Relationships with Outside Professionals

To effectively treat those with co-occurring disorders, programs are encouraged to provide services in as close to an integrated approach as possible. AOS or MHOS programs can build upon their existing treatment services by developing standard protocols and defined relationships with other local service providers. The AOS program can team up with an outside mental health service provider, while the MHOS program can team up with an outside addiction treatment provider. Integrated treatment can happen when these teams work together to determine how to handle transfers and referrals and to discuss plans for common patients.

Billing Mechanisms

What are your program's billing mechanisms for mental health services? Do they support or inhibit treatment for co-occurring problems? Some addiction treatment programs can only receive reimbursement for services provided to those with substance use disorders; they may not receive reimbursement for providing mental health services. Some mental health programs can only receive payment for services provided to those with psychiatric disorders; no payment may be accepted for addiction treatment. Providing adequate treatment for those with co-occurring disorders is very difficult and cumbersome for these types of programs.

Programs that can receive reimbursement for both addiction treatment and mental health services have a much greater capacity to serve those with co-occurring disorders. The agency director or other top-level financial personnel (such as the chief financial officer) should be knowledgeable about this information.

Evaluate Your Billing Mechanisms

To analyze your program's financial structure, assess your program's source of funding and determine if your organization receives reimbursement for providing services for both substance use disorders and psychiatric disorders.

Improve Your Billing Mechanisms

Addiction treatment programs have enhanced their performance on this benchmark through two primary strategies. The first, and perhaps most obvious, is the pursuit

---

Evaluate an Addiction or Mental Health Treatment Program

*In general, the **financial structure** of an AOS or MHOS program
falls into one of these four categories.*

The program

- accepts payment for services provided to individuals with a primary substance use disorder. There is no reimbursement for services provided to treat psychiatric disorders.

- accepts payment for services provided to treat mental health and substance use disorders, but the patient must have a substance use disorder. The staff and administrators believe there are barriers to reimbursement for mental health services.

- accepts payment for services provided to treat mental health and substance use disorders, but the patient must have a substance use disorder.

- accepts payment for services provided to treat both mental health and substance use disorders equally. Reimbursement is not dependent on the patient having a substance use disorder.

---

of licensure and certification from a regulatory agency such that mental health or addiction treatment services can be funded. This often involves a longer-term process, including extensive applications, changes in a variety of other policies, shifts in human resources, and other changes. Another strategy, which requires less change than agency licensure does, is developing a mechanism to bill on behalf of staff or contractors with mental health licensure. This includes physicians, psychologists, social workers, and licensed mental health counselors. This enables the unbundling of services and additional services to be covered.

A program that cannot receive reimbursement for both mental health and addiction treatment services will be discouraged to provide integrated treatment for both disorders. Programs with these types of financial constraints have a few options. The program can locate physicians or prescribers on whose behalf they can bill for unbundled services. Another approach is to obtain contract or grant funding to provide adjunctive pharmacological or psychosocial services. Taking this step will help move an AOS or MHOS program to the DDC level.

Programs at the DDE level do not have these same kind of financial constraints because they are able to bill Medicaid, Medicare, or other third-party insurance that do not require distinctions between patients with psychiatric disorders and substance use disorders. Because these organizations can bill for both types of services, they can provide both types of services and therefore provide comprehensive treatment to those with co-occurring disorders.

After evaluating your program's structure, proceed to chapter 5 where you will inspect your program milieu and culture to get an idea of the perception persons with co-occurring disorders, and the general community, have when they are exposed to advertising and other media about your program. This includes messages patients receive when they enter your program's waiting room and clinical areas.

•   •   •

Policy: Evaluating Your Program Milieu

Once you have evaluated the program structure that your organization operates within, you will begin to inspect your program milieu to assess the treatment culture that is communicated to the general community and to patients. This includes looking at advertising and other media messages about your program.

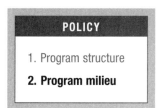

It also involves determining the explicit and implicit messages patients receive—via staff attitudes and by looking at materials such as educational posters or brochures—when they enter your program waiting room or are in clinical areas.

Understanding Your Program Milieu

The program milieu encompasses the physical and social environment within which patients receive services. This environment has both tangible and intangible characteristics.

Tangible characteristics of your program can be observed through direct observation. These include program information materials for patients, which can be in the form of posters on walls, brochures found in waiting rooms, and materials given to patients and families to educate them about co-occurring disorders or about any specific illnesses for which they are receiving treatment.

The intangible characteristics of your program include the "feeling" or ambiance of a program. Patients may wonder: Is this the sort of place where any problem can be raised? Is this the sort of place where I may be discriminated against or be discharged if I reveal psychiatric symptoms, or even a history of having symptoms? Only a patient who receives services can tell you about these issues. Frontline clinical staff may have one attitude toward mental health or substance use disorders; receptionists, residential program aides, or even the housekeeping staff may have different attitudes that convey acceptance or discrimination.

Your program milieu communicates to patients what is acceptable and what is not. Certain programs foster an ambiance that assures patients that both addiction and mental health issues are okay to bring up and that treatment is

```
┌─────────────────────────────────────────┐
│        PROGRAM MILIEU BENCHMARKS          │
│                                           │
│ Program milieu refers to two specific     │
│ benchmarks:                               │
│          1. Program environment           │
│          2. Program literature            │
└─────────────────────────────────────────┘
```

offered for both. This open environment allows patients to bring up an addiction or a mental health issue during a therapy session. The materials in your organization's brochure racks should not only include information about Twelve Step and peer recovery support group meetings that are available in the neighboring community, tips for escaping domestic violence, and options for treating sexually transmitted diseases, but also information about the most common co-occurring psychiatric disorders.

Utilize the Perspective of Patients

Patients in integrated co-occurring treatment programs often cannot define the program as an addiction treatment or mental health program. Instead they may describe the range of addiction and mental health topics that are discussed and treated. For example, a bipolar alcoholic patient in a DDE program may understand that the bipolar disorder is as important to deal with as addiction to alcohol. This person will describe how the treatment program helps treat both mental health and substance use disorders and how both are important for recovery.

In contrast, a patient in an AOS program may describe a stigma associated with having a mental health disorder or with taking a medication to address it. This patient may feel less adequate than people who do not require prescription medications. He or she may feel shame, as if he or she is taking the easier, softer way because of the need for medication for a co-occurring psychiatric disorder.

Similarly, a patient in an MHOS program may feel a stigma associated with having an addiction to cocaine, alcohol, or another drug, in addition to a mental health disorder. This patient may feel shame about alcohol or other drug use, which complicates treatment for either disorder. This patient may feel that the clinician treats him or her as a bad or untrustworthy person, or that he or she may be seen as weak or lacking the willpower to stop drinking or using.

Remember that some patients will experience a differential or equivalent degree of stigma and/or acceptability in having both an addictive and psychiatric disorder, regardless of the supportiveness of the program environment.

In the sections that follow, the two program milieu benchmarks are defined in detail, and examples of programs that are operating at DDC and DDE levels are given. Suggestions for how a program may consider enhancing its performance on each benchmark are also noted.

Program Environment

Does your program expect and welcome the treatment of both mental health and substance-related disorders? Benchmark 1 (program environment) reflects the more intangible cultural dimension that evaluates whether patients with all types or levels of co-occurring disorders feel welcomed and confident about the treatment options offered at your facility.

Evaluate Your Program Environment

When you observe your organization's environment and conduct interviews with staff and patients, it is not difficult to determine if persons with co-occurring disorders are welcome in your facility. This investigation may also reveal how your organization's treatment policies and values are communicated in posters, pamphlets, and other supporting documents that patients are exposed to. Staff attitudes and behaviors, as well as the program's mission statement and values, must also be taken into consideration.

Evaluate an Addiction Treatment Program

*In general, the **environment** of an addiction treatment program may fall into one of these five categories.*

The program

- focuses on individuals with substance use disorders only. Individuals with psychiatric disorders are not welcomed or treated, which can lead them to repress or deny concerns about either disorder.

- expects to treat only individuals with substance use disorders, but, depending on the clinicians' preferences, this program does not always reject individuals with psychiatric disorders. There are no formal guidelines or documentation of acceptance or refusal based on mental health conditions.

- focuses primarily on individuals with substance use disorders, but the program is willing and able to accept individuals with mild or stable forms of co-occurring mental health disorders. This is reflected in the program's documentation.

- expects and treats individuals with co-occurring disorders regardless of severity, but has informal procedures and protocols for doing so. There is no supporting documentation to reflect this service.

- routinely accepts individuals with co-occurring disorders regardless of severity and has formally mandated this aspect of its service through its mission statement, philosophy, welcoming policy, and appropriate protocols.

Perhaps the most important source of information on this issue comes from the patients and families themselves. Try conducting focus groups, individual "exit" interviews, or casual conversations with patients. When patients are told they are "consumers" and see that you are interested in their opinion, most are willing to discuss their likes and dislikes, or at least offer recommendations. Another approach is the ethnographic technique of "walk-thru" methodology. This involves having an unbiased actor attend your program with both a mental health and a substance use disorder in order to gather data on the patient experience, including how the staff respond. Walk-thru methods are regaining popularity but may pose ethical considerations.

Improve Your Program Environment

AOS programs focus primarily on treating individuals with substance use disorders and are neither open nor explicit about acknowledging or treating a co-occurring psychiatric disorder. Because this type of discussion is not encouraged, patients

---

Evaluate a Mental Health Treatment Program

*In general, the **environment** of a mental health treatment program may fall into one of these five categories.*

The program

- focuses on individuals with mental health disorders only. Individuals with substance use disorders are not welcomed or treated, which can lead them to repress or deny concerns about either disorder.

- expects to treat only individuals with mental health disorders, but, depending on the clinicians' preferences, this program does not always reject individuals with substance use disorders. There are no formal guidelines or documentation of acceptance or refusal based on the level of substance use.

- focuses primarily on individuals with mental health disorders, but the program is willing and able to accept individuals with mild or stable forms of co-occurring substance use disorders. This is reflected in the program's documentation.

- expects and treats individuals with co-occurring disorders regardless of severity, but has informal procedures and protocols for doing so. There is no supporting documentation to reflect this service.

- routinely accepts individuals with co-occurring disorders regardless of severity and has formally mandated this aspect of its service through its mission statement, philosophy, welcoming policy, and appropriate protocols.

---

may not feel that they can ask for assistance with a mental health disorder at the same time. In a similar way, MHOS programs do not typically encourage or promote a dialogue about substance use disorders. These patients may feel ashamed or too inhibited to discuss a challenging substance use disorder, even when it is complicating their mental health treatment.

An AOS or MHOS program can move up to the DDC level by changing its environment to demonstrate that it is welcoming and accepting of persons with co-occurring disorders. This can occur by making brochures and literature about various psychiatric disorders readily available in waiting areas. A program can host community meetings, family visits, or other sessions that educate patients, patients' families, and the larger community on the best treatment for co-occurring disorders. In this type of program environment, individuals with co-occurring disorders may feel more "normal" and more able to discuss comprehensive treatment options with an addiction treatment or mental health care professional.

To move to the DDE level, programs must show equal focus on addiction and psychiatric disorders. A patient in this type of program is encouraged to discuss and seek treatment for both addiction and psychiatric disorders and is not made to feel inferior. Typically, this patient can state that he or she has a co-occurring disorder, or two (or more) disorders, and can discuss the treatment plan for both (or all) disorders. This patient may comment that this is the first program that has addressed both disorders at the same time.

Program Literature

In your program, what types of advertising, media, and patient education materials are distributed, and do they reflect a focus on co-occurring disorders? By walking around the waiting room and clinical therapy areas of a treatment facility, it's fairly easy to determine if the program addresses both mental health and substance use disorders. It's important to examine these waiting areas and other common areas for patients and families in order to evaluate the types of literature and educational materials that are available to patients. When examining your program milieu, it's also important to look at advertising and other media messages that communicate your program's identity to patients and to the general community.

Evaluate Your Program Literature

The type of media and patient education materials displayed and distributed by your organization is a clear indication of the types of services provided and the diversity of individuals treated. Typically, AOS programs display only materials related to drug and alcohol problems with the occasional brochure featuring sexually transmitted diseases or substance use during pregnancy. To move up to the DDC level, an addiction treatment program can provide and distribute patient education materials on co-occurring disorders or specific common disorders such as depression, anxiety, and post-traumatic stress disorder (PTSD).

Similarly a MHOS program may only display materials related to mental health problems. To move to the DDC level, MHOS programs can provide information on alcohol and drug use problems, information on peer recovery support groups (such as a list of AA and NA meetings), or any material that could reduce stigma for substance use issues.

Evaluate an Addiction Treatment Program

When you evaluate the physical and social setting of an addiction treatment program, you may find that the organization's **media and patient education materials** address

- only substance use disorders
- both substance use and mental health disorders, but the mental health materials are not routinely accessible or displayed
- both substance use and mental health disorders
- both substance use and mental health disorders and also co-occurring disorder–specific concerns, such as the effects of co-occurring disorders on psychological function, health, and success in attending peer recovery support group meetings, and medications versus drugs and coordinating services with multiple providers

---

Evaluate a Mental Health Treatment Program

When you evaluate the physical and social setting of a mental health treatment program, you may find that the organization's **media and patient education materials** address

- only mental health disorders
- both mental health and substance use disorders, but the addiction treatment materials are not routinely accessible or displayed
- both mental health and substance use disorders
- both mental health and substance use disorders and also co-occurring disorder–specific concerns, such as the effects of co-occurring disorders on psychological function, health, and success in attending peer recovery support group meetings, and medications versus drugs and coordinating services with multiple providers

Patient Education Materials

A complete set of Fact Sheets on common co-occurring disorders is available in curricula ❷, ❸, and ❺ of this Co-occurring Disorders Program. These Fact Sheets discuss the following topics:

- general information on co-occurring disorders
- bipolar disorder
- dysthymia
- generalized anxiety disorder
- major depression
- obsessive-compulsive disorder (OCD)
- panic disorder
- post-traumatic stress disorder (PTSD)
- schizophrenia
- schizoaffective disorder
- social anxiety disorder

The Substance Abuse and Mental Health Services Administration (SAMHSA) and the National Institute of Mental Health (NIMH) Web sites, and other professional organizations including the American Psychiatric Association and American Psychological Association, also produce educational materials. See the CD-ROM ▢ included with this guidebook for a link to these sites.

A diverse mix of materials for patients and family members is included in the Co-occurring Disorders Program. The program DVD, *A Guide for Living with Co-occurring Disorders,* is also an excellent educational resource for patients and families.

Educational videos on co-occurring disorders are also available from Hazelden Publishing. These resources can serve to systematically raise awareness and promote discussion during treatment groups and family education or visit programs, and result in educated consumers of addiction treatment services. For a list of Hazelden products on co-occurring disorders, see the CD-ROM ▢ included with this guidebook.

Improve Your Program Environment

To move to DDE level, a program must show that substance use and psychiatric disorders are treated equally. One way this can happen is through equitable availability and distribution of materials on both disorders. For example, a program at this level should help individuals develop realistic expectations about their prospects for recovery by discussing the possibility of co-occurring disorders and by explaining how frequently individuals with substance use disorders also have depression, bipolar disorder, anxiety disorders, and PTSD. Programs should also describe the differences between drugs and medications, the difficulties and challenges of living with co-occurring disorders, and the possibility of seeking help through peer recovery support groups and meetings.

• • •

Clinical Practice: Evaluating Screening and Assessment Procedures

CHAPTER 6

Most treatment professionals consider clinical practice to be the most central issue that must be evaluated and often improved to expand an organization's capacity to offer integrated treatment for people with co-occurring disorders. Clinical practice is affected by three primary components: assessment, treatment, and continuity of care. This chapter will evaluate *assessment* as an important

CLINICAL PRACTICE

3. Assessment

4. Treatment

5. Continuity of care

part of clinical practice. Chapter 7 will detail how a program can evaluate and improve the *treatment* process of clinical practice. Chapter 8 will complete the analysis of clinical practice by explaining the importance of *continuity of care* in treating people with co-occurring disorders.

This chapter covers patient assessment, which is chronologically the first step in the clinical process, followed by treatment (covered in chapter 7), and last by continuity of care (covered in chapter 8). These three dimensions form the core of a program's treatment approach and constitute twenty-two of thirty-five DDCAT benchmark items. In other words, roughly two-thirds of the program assessment benchmarks fall in the clinical practice domain.

In the sections that follow, each of the seven assessment benchmarks are defined in detail, and examples of programs that are operating at DDC and DDE levels are given. Suggestions for how a program may consider enhancing its performance on each benchmark are also noted.

Curriculum ❶ *Screening and Assessment,* if utilized, will provide the treatment program all the necessary measures to achieve DDC- or DDE-level performance on the assessment practice benchmarks.

Understanding Your Program's Assessment Practices

When evaluating each of these aspects of the clinical practices of your program, consider how consistently these practices occur from clinician to clinician, and from patient to patient. In other words, is there consistency in these practices and are they routine? One simple way to think about this question is to ask yourself, "Is this assessment practice consistent because it is driven by a systematic protocol or does it occur only at the discretion of each individual clinician on each day?" That is, is the practice clinician-driven or protocol-driven? Programs must consider these potential variations at the front end of treatment and how they may alter a particular patient's treatment experience.

ASSESSMENT BENCHMARKS

Assessment refers to seven specific benchmarks that should be evaluated in this order:

1. Screening

2. Assessment

3. Diagnosis

4. Differential diagnosis

5. Program acceptance based on acuity

6. Program acceptance based on severity

7. Assessment of patient motivation and preference

The intent here is the reduction of variability in patient care from clinician to clinician or perhaps from program to program. Although enormous variability exists in all health services, from orthopedics to cardiovascular care, both addiction treatment and mental health treatment specialties are striving to reduce this variation by working toward greater systematization and precision. This is not meant to minimize the significant role of the relationship between clinician and patient, or reduce the value of clinical judgment to robot mechanics. It is meant to promote systematic approaches that can reduce significant variability in practice and outcomes, and still engage the intimately personal, if not craftlike, application of skills by individual clinicians.

A story at an addiction treatment program may illustrate this point:

> Joan, an addiction treatment clinician, recently attended a weekend workshop on women who suffer from addiction and trauma. On her first week back in the office, she was exquisitely tuned in to the traumatic backgrounds of the seven patients who were scheduled for intake. She was careful in inquiring and probing about the patients' traumatic life events, and she even applied her knowledge to ask about re-experiencing, avoidance, and hyperarousal symptoms to see if any of the patients had PTSD symptoms. All but one of the patients Joan assessed that week received a "rule out" diagnosis of PTSD.

Bill, an addiction treatment clinician at the same organization, was unable to attend the workshop Joan experienced. Bill also conducted seven patient intakes on the same day. None of the intakes Bill conducted that day, or that month, received a diagnosis of PTSD.

The point of these two stories is to show how an educational workshop on mental health issues likely enhanced Joan's ability to screen for PTSD. After months or years have passed, will Joan assess patients with this same level of purposeful inquiry? What about the screening practices of Bill, who had not been exposed to recent training? These two clinicians work for the same organization and yet their screening methods are not consistent.

Screening

Patient screenings are typically conducted at the time a patient presents for services, or in some cases by phone even before a patient presents at your physical location. Screening is used to determine the possibility of a co-occurring substance use or psychiatric disorder; it is not meant to determine definitively that a person does have a psychiatric or substance use disorder, nor does it identify specific types of disorders.

What are your organization's screening practices? Screening can be seen as the radar system of an addiction or mental health treatment program. It is an attempt to systematically detect the presence or absence of a psychiatric or substance use problem. For example, most patients who present for addiction treatment will also report anxiety symptoms. The anxiety may be associated with intoxication, withdrawal, or craving. The anxiety may also be associated with current life circumstances—such as divorce, job loss, legal concerns, or an awareness of medical problems—that leave the person feeling fearful and unsettled. The anxiety may also be associated with making a change in substance use ("How can I possibly survive without using?"), or the likelihood of treatment success ("How can these people possibly help me?"). The anxiety may also be associated with an anxiety disorder, such as a generalized anxiety disorder, panic disorder, or social phobia, as defined in the *DSM-IV*. The anxiety may also be associated with PTSD.

Screening is the beginning of the process; it is not a diagnosis. Screening indicates the likelihood of a disorder that meets or exceeds the threshold of symptoms for a clinical diagnosis. Screening must be verified by an objective assessment in order to verify a clinical diagnosis. If a patient's mental health or substance use disorder is missed by a clinician, his or her overall treatment outcome will likely be worse than if all mental health or substance use disorders were assessed and treated.

In some programs, screening takes on the format of "screening out" people with certain kinds of disorders. Certain symptoms and histories are flags that the patient is not appropriate for a program that treats non-severe mental illness. This type of patient will be referred to another program, or in some cases, simply denied further access to this program's intake services. For example, a person who is diagnosed with severe mental illness (such as schizophrenia) or is suicidal and requires immediate medical supervision will be referred elsewhere.

Many agencies rely on these questions for mental health screening:

- Have you ever been diagnosed with or treated for a mental health problem?
- Are you now or have you ever taken any medications for a mental health problem?
- Have you ever been hospitalized for psychiatric reasons?

Some agencies include a blank section under "psychological/psychiatric" on a "biopsychosocial" intake screening form for writing open-ended notes about the patient.

Implementing Collaborative Referral Procedures

Some AOS or MHOS programs, due to capacity, staffing, and financial circumstances, may only aspire to screen for co-occurring disorders and not deliver treatments for mental health and substance use disorders. This type of program would need to implement standard collaborative referral and linkage procedures.

The screening, brief intervention, and referral to treatment (SBIRT) model has been found effective in primary health care settings in reducing substance-related problems and depression, either via brief intervention or more effective linkage to other providers.

For more information about SBIRT, visit http://sbirt.samhsa.gov. A link to this Web site is provided on the CD-ROM that accompanies this guidebook.

Although this type of questioning is common and quick, it is likely unreliable in obtaining useful data for screening purposes. Many addiction treatment providers are interested in acquiring and using standardized screening measures for the most common psychiatric problems that occur with substance use, such as depression, anxiety, PTSD, and social phobia. There are also some general screening measures for a broader range of psychiatric problems (including bipolar disorder and psychotic spectrum disorders).

Evaluate Patient Symptoms

There has been historical mistrust of self-report measures in addiction treatment programs, largely driven by the expectation that patients will minimize or deny the presence of substance use problems. There is no evidence suggesting that patients are unreliable in self-reporting of psychiatric symptoms, but there are some inherent threats to accurate reporting. These include a clinician's subjective interpretation of patient responses and patients that exaggerate their psychiatric symptoms. Nonetheless, patient self-report measures are a useful and cost-effective tool for systematically determining the likely presence of a psychiatric disorder. They continue to be underutilized probably out of historical bias and fear of the findings: "If we know there is a problem we'll have to do something about it." (This is another version of "Don't ask; don't tell.")

If the screening measure is negative, it could mean that there are no symptoms and no disorders. It could also mean that a patient is mistrustful. Many programs repeat the screening once the patient has settled into a more trusting relationship with clinicians. It is also possible that some symptoms will not emerge until after a period of abstinence. These symptoms may also be detected by readministering the screening measure.

Positive screening responses must also be interpreted by a clinician. In methadone clinics some patients report symptoms in an attempt to be medicated sooner or at higher doses. Other reasons for inaccurate positive responses include substance-related factors (withdrawal, intoxication, or craving), treatment-related factors (more symptoms, more help), and stressful life-situation factors (divorce, loss of job).

Improve Accurate Identification of People with Disorders

Using standardized assessment measuring tools can reduce clinician variability in detecting the potential presence of a psychiatric disorder or substance use disorder. This increases the systematic identification of persons suffering from one or more disorders. Some programs only use screening measures when they suspect that a patient has a problem. Unfortunately, this type of reactive approach often only identifies people with obvious problems, and it often fails to identify people who suffer from less severe conditions.

People will often reveal psychological concerns when they report on a computer or on a paper-and-pencil survey. Some studies have actually found that many people are more likely to disclose mental health or substance use issues to inanimate modalities than they are to a trained clinical interviewer.

When you develop a systematic screening protocol for your program, you

1. systemize the intake and admission process;

2. provide a common language and an objective metric;

3. provide staff with a valid measuring instrument;

4. facilitate consistent training;

5. improve the validity of patient outcome measurement.

Evaluate Your Screening Process

To evaluate your current screening processes, begin by conducting interviews with clinicians and reviewing the medical records or intake screening packets your program uses to determine if your program routinely and systematically screens for both substance use and psychiatric disorders.

Evaluate an Addiction Treatment Program

*In general, the **assessment practices** of an addiction treatment program may fall into one of these four categories.*

The program

■ does not conduct any screenings for psychiatric disorders, unless it is the clinician's preference to do so.

■ conducts basic screenings for psychiatric problems, which might include a review of symptoms, treatment history, current medications, and/or suicide/homicide history; however, these screenings are not part of the program's standard protocols and do not occur with any regularity. The results of the screenings often vary based on individual clinicians.

■ routinely conducts screenings for psychiatric problems using a standard set of questions or items as part of protocol.

■ routinely conducts systematic screenings for both substance use and psychiatric disorders using standardized, reliable, and validated instrument(s). These screenings are vital components in determining the treatment plan.

Improve Your Screening Process

Programs may conduct screenings to determine whether a patient has a co-occurring psychiatric disorder. At the most basic level, AOS programs typically ask basic questions about current and past medication use, prior psychiatric hospitalizations, and if the patient has ever been diagnosed with a mental health disorder. These screenings vary based on the clinician conducting them. The same is true of MHOS programs, which may or may not ask about substance use, depending on the clinician performing the assessment. To move to the DDC level, these programs can standardize screening questions and incorporate screenings into the standard intake protocols or treatment protocols.

To move to the DDE level, DDC programs must institute standardized screening measures for mental health and substance use disorders. These measures can assess for more general psychiatric symptoms and are sensitive to identifying psychiatric problems. Examples of some general measures include the Modified Mini Screen (MMS) or the Global Appraisal of Individual Needs (GAIN) Short Screener (GAIN-SS). Measures with greater specificity to screen for the most prevalent disorders are also recommended. These may include measures for depression (e.g., Beck Depression Inventory), anxiety (e.g., Beck Anxiety Inventory), PTSD (e.g., PTSD Checklist), and social phobia (e.g., Social Interaction Anxiety Scale).

Evaluate a Mental Health Treatment Program

*In general, the **assessment practices** of a mental health treatment program may fall into one of these four categories.*

The program

- does not conduct any screenings for substance use disorders, unless it is the clinician's preference to do so.

- conducts basic screenings for substance use disorders, which might include a review of symptoms, addiction treatment history, current medications, and/or substance use history; however, these screenings are not part of the program's standard protocols and do not occur with any regularity. The results of the screenings often vary based on individual clinicians.

- routinely conducts screenings for substance use disorders using a standard set of questions or items as part of the protocol.

- routinely conducts systematic screenings for both substance use and psychiatric disorders using standardized, reliable, and validated instrument(s). These screenings are vital components in determining the treatment plan. Some providers at this level use objective toxicological tests for the presence of substances in urine, breath, or blood samples.

Curriculum ❶ *Screening and Assessment* helps clinicians accurately and systematically evaluate patients before treatment options are addressed. Included are specific measures for screening, assessment, and differential diagnostics, and tools to identify the patient's stage of motivation. Selecting screening measures is an important process. Measures themselves vary in terms of relevance, length, and time to complete. They also vary in reliability, validity, and cost. *Screening and Assessment* will guide you through this process.

> For more information on screening, see SAMHSA's Co-Occurring Center for Excellence (COCE) paper called *Screening, Assessment, and Treatment Planning for Persons with Co-Occurring Disorders* available online at www.coce.samhsa.gov.
>
> See the CD-ROM included with this guidebook for a direct link to the paper.

Assessment

Are your assessment practices systematic and protocol-driven? A systematic, protocol-driven approach is important in each of the three clinical practice benchmarks (assessment, treatment, and continuity of care), but is most important in patient assessment. Assessment generally begins when a patient first presents to a clinician at an addiction treatment center or a mental health center. The attending clinician asks the patient probing questions to reveal any disorders that exist. If a clinician finds evidence of a mental health or substance use disorder, more specific questions are asked to explore the potential for one or more disorders.

Given the overlap between and among mental health and substance use disorders, a clinician must take pains to examine the timing and sequence of a patient's symptoms to evaluate whether or not a mental health and substance use disorder exist independently from each other. At this time, the clinician must decide whether, based on the nature and/or severity of the disorder (or disorders), the patient can be accepted for treatment into the program. At the same time, the clinician should also estimate the patient's motivation and/or interest in participating in treatment. (Refer to the clinician's guide of curriculum ❶ *Screening and Assessment,* which has standardized measures to assess patient motivation for both addiction and mental health treatment.)

Evaluate Your Assessment Process

What are your organization's assessment practices? Does your program conduct routine assessments after a positive screening for psychiatric symptoms? Screening will detect the potential presence of a disorder. An assessment process will verify it. Much like a radar system that is not always able to distinguish between a small missile and a large flock of geese, screening alone may not provide a complete picture of the health of a patient. An assessment by an addiction treatment clinician will be necessary to determine the presence of a mental health disorder (distinct from substance-induced symptoms), current life stressors, and reactions to the demands of addiction treatment. In a similar way, a mental health clinician will need to perform an assessment to determine if a substance use disorder exists, in addition to a mental health disorder.

The most common approach to assessment for mental health problems in addiction treatment programs is the "biopsychosocial" assessment form completed by an addiction clinician. Though many clinicians can use this form to assess and probe for a variety of psychiatric disorders, most do not. Structured assessment measures such as the Mini International Neuropsychiatric Interview (MINI) 5.0, GAIN, or the Structured Clinical Interview for DSM-IV (SCID) can help guide a trained clinician to identify many psychiatric disorders; however, these standard measures are often too costly to implement and are seen by many agencies as primarily research-driven. The Addiction Severity Index (ASI) is a more user-friendly assessment of substance use problems including psychiatric, social/family, medical, legal, and work functioning. The ASI is widely used but is more a measure of severity than of psychiatric conditions. Therefore, aside from GAIN, there is no currently valid, useful, and systematic approach to assessing for both substance use and psychiatric disorders or problems.

For more information about structured assessment measures visit these sites:

- Global Appraisal of Individual Needs (GAIN): www.chestnut.org

- The Structured Clinical Interview for DSM-IV (SCID): www.scid4.org

- Mini International Neuropsychiatric Interview (MINI) 5.0:
  www.medical-outcomes.com/HTMLFiles/MINI/MINI_FAQs.htm
  For direct links to these sites, see the ⬛ CD-ROM that accompanies this guidebook.

The best approach often involves having a licensed or competent clinician review the screening measure information with the patient, followed by using the *DSM-IV* criteria to more thoroughly evaluate the potential for a psychiatric disorder.

A growing number of programs have implemented or are in the process of adopting electronic medical records (EMR). At the time of this printing, no commercial EMR products are available that adequately assess for co-occurring psychiatric disorders. Some providers have customized their own EMR versions so that co-occurring disorders can be reviewed and listed as problems.

Improve Your Assessment Process

Assessments are used to establish or rule out co-occurring disorders. In addition, assessments may also be used to determine a patient's strengths or problem areas that may affect treatment and recovery. It is common for the outcome of an assessment to be a formal diagnosis of a mental health or substance use disorder, but such a diagnosis is not required.

Programs at the AOS level can move to the DDC level by offering on-site mental health assessments routinely and consistently. Programs at the DDC level can move to the DDE level by establishing a systemic procedure for conducting mental health assessments for all individuals. These assessments must be standardized

---

Evaluate an Addiction or Mental Health Treatment Program

*In general, an AOS or MHOS program's **clinical practice assessment** may fall into one of these four categories.*

The program

- does not conduct an assessment for both psychiatric and substance use disorders when screening indicates the possibility of co-occurring disorders. Instead, the program may monitor for these disorders, but only to determine whether or not they can provide services to the patient.

- does not conduct an assessment for both psychiatric and substance use disorders as standard protocol upon a positive screening, but may do so based on clinician preference and expertise.

- does not conduct formal assessments for psychiatric and substance use disorders on-site as is necessary based on a positive screen. These types of assessments can only be conducted by a competent provider who, by education, training, licensure, certification, or supervised experience, is capable of conducting the evaluation for both types of disorders.

- routinely conducts standardized and formal integrated assessments on all individuals for both substance use and psychiatric disorders.

and retrieve the same information regardless of the person conducting the assessment. This can either be accomplished by an electronic medical record (EMR) or a semi-structured clinical interview (GAIN, MINI 5.0, ASI, SCID), or another well-defined and thorough protocol developed by the program. Refer to curriculum ❶ *Screening and Assessment,* which provides assessment instruments that would enable a program to move from an AOS or MHOS level to a DDC level, or from DDC to DDE on this benchmark.

Diagnosis

Does your program make and document psychiatric and substance use diagnoses? Diagnosis is important because, although inexact, the presence of a disorder (versus a symptom) is often an indication for additional treatment. For example, screening indicated that Steve, a patient, had severe symptoms of depression and a probable mood disorder. An assessment revealed that Steve was in fact experiencing depressive symptoms. Further, the assessment revealed that Steve had a positive family history for depression (his father), suffered severe depression during a two-year period when he abstained from cocaine and alcohol (his drugs of choice), and two months after the most recent treatment episode, Steve was still struggling with these symptoms. The clinician accurately assessed that Steve suffers from an independent mood disorder (versus a substance-induced mood disorder). However, the clinician neither diagnosed nor documented Steve's substance use. For this reason, the chances for Steve receiving integrated mental health and addiction treatment are significantly diminished.

Enhanced programs routinely follow the process from screening to assessment to diagnosis so that information about a patient's co-occurring disorder is not lost but tracked through this important phase of treatment.

Evaluate Your Diagnostic Process
After addressing screening and assessment procedures, look at your organization's use of diagnostic nomenclature when identifying and specifying that a patient has a particular psychiatric or substance use disorder. In some cases, problems are screened as positive, and a formal assessment is then conducted to determine the presence of a particular disorder. More often, the disorder is not formally diagnosed, recorded, or noted as "ruled out." This may happen if the clinician doing the assessment is not licensed or certified to offer both substance use and psychiatric diagnoses.

Improve Your Diagnostic Process

Depending on a program's capacity, diagnostic assessments for psychiatric disorders may not accompany assessments for substance use disorders. In order for an AOS program to move to the DDC level, it must follow the standard processes of screening, assessment, and then formal diagnosis. Simply registering or ruling out a psychiatric disorder is not sufficient for the DDC level. To move to the DDE level, these diagnostic assessments, when present, are specific and may include all five of the axes on the *DSM-IV* multi-axial system.

For more information on diagnosis of co-occurring substance use and psychiatric disorders, refer to curriculum ❶ *Screening and Assessment,* which provides the necessary instruments to ascertain and distinguish both types of diagnoses.

Evaluate an Addiction Treatment Program

In general, addiction treatment programs' assessment criteria vary and some programs may

- focus solely on diagnosing substance use disorders, while diagnosing psychiatric disorders may even be discouraged or not recorded.
- occasionally provide diagnostic assessments of psychiatric disorders on an as-needed basis, but capacity to do so is limited.
- regularly provide and document mental health disorders; however, the diagnostic assessments are inconsistent depending on the program's capacity.
- regularly conduct standard, formal, and comprehensive diagnostic assessments; therefore, mental health disorders are consistently identified and documented.

Evaluate a Mental Health Treatment Program

In general, mental health treatment programs' assessment criteria vary and some programs may

- focus solely on diagnosing mental health disorders, while diagnosing substance use disorders may even be discouraged or not recorded.
- occasionally provide diagnoses of substance use disorders on an as-needed basis, but capacity to do so is limited.
- regularly provide and document diagnoses of substance use disorders; however, the diagnostic assessments are inconsistent depending on the program's capacity.
- regularly conduct standard, formal, and comprehensive diagnostic assessments; therefore, substance use disorders are consistently identified and documented.

Differential Diagnosis

Do your program's medical records include psychiatric and substance use history? The most common substance-induced mental health disorders are mood and anxiety disorders. Although the *DSM-IV* provides some guidance in criteria to make the distinction between substance-induced and independent psychiatric disorders, the specifications are imprecise. To conclusively make the distinction, or to make it with some degree of confidence, utilize reassessments over predetermined intervals of time. With reassessment, particularly after periods of abstinence from alcohol and other drugs, the most accurate diagnostic impressions are likely formed. Curriculum ❶ *Screening and Assessment* will help clinicians at your organization make this differentiation.

Evaluate Your Differential Diagnosis Process

In many patients the onset of a mental health disorder and substance use disorder is simultaneous. Many have never had a period of abstinence for more than thirty days, and the "end of withdrawal" in many patients is complicated by the type of drug used, such as opioids or cocaine, which can present protracted withdrawal syndromes. The Clinical Institute for Withdrawal Assessment Scale (included in curriculum ❶ *Screening and Assessment*) will help clinicians identify common withdrawal signs and symptoms. The final clinical recourse is to carefully monitor and reassess these symptoms in the present treatment episode to best make the differential diagnosis.

The degree to which this is accomplished, and the extent to which it is done in a systematic and routine manner, tells how enhanced a program's services are for its patients with co-occurring disorders. See curriculum ❶ *Screening and Assessment* for help with this practice.

Improve Your Differential Diagnosis Process

To provide enhanced services for individuals with co-occurring disorders, a program must routinely collect information about both mental health disorders and substance use histories, as well as information regarding the interaction of the disorders. This information should be routinely documented in medical records for all patients. It is important to note that, in some instances, assessing and diagnosing psychiatric disorders in addiction treatment may be complicated by the effects of substances, from intoxication to craving to withdrawal to protracted withdrawal. The *DSM-IV* provides some guidelines in making differential diagnosis (substance-induced versus independent disorders). The Clinical Institute for Withdrawal Assessment Scale (CIWA) assists in identifying the type and severity of withdrawal symptoms. See curriculum ❶ *Screening and Assessment* for additional assistance.

For an AOS or MHOS level program to move to the DDC level, the program should document information about ages of onset for disorders, periods of active

---

Evaluate an Addiction Treatment Program

In general, an addiction treatment program's **differential diagnosis** assessment criteria do one of the following:

- focus solely on routinely collecting information about substance use history, not mental health history.

- encourage the collection of mental health history in an unstructured and undefined manner. Individual clinicians determine what information to gather and how to record it. In other cases, the program follows a standard procedure for gathering mental health history but does not collect it with regularity.

- routinely collect and record both substance use and mental health history.

- routinely collect both mental health and substance use histories as part of the standard and systematic assessment process. In addition, information regarding the interaction of the disorders is recorded.

Evaluate a Mental Health Treatment Program

In general, a mental health treatment program's **differential diagnosis** assessment criteria do one of the following:

- focus solely on routinely collecting information about mental health history, not substance use history.

- encourage the collection of substance use history in an unstructured and undefined manner. Individual clinicians determine what information to gather and how to record it. In other cases, the program follows a standard procedure for gathering a substance use history but does not collect it with regularity.

- routinely collect and record both mental health and substance use history.

- routinely collect both substance use and mental health histories as part of the standard and systematic assessment process. In addition, information regarding the interaction of the disorders is recorded.

---

substance use or abstinence, as well as the course of the substance use during treatment or remission of the psychiatric disorder. To move to the DDE level, the complexity of the interaction of the disorders must be documented and recognized in a formal manner on all medical records. Timeline follow-back (TLFB) calendars are helpful tools for keeping track of this information.

Program Acceptance Based on Acuity

Is patient acceptance in your program based on the level of psychiatric symptom acuity? Addiction treatment and mental health programs cannot entirely avoid or deflect persons with co-occurring disorders. The loose telephone screening or "screening out" questions have only a reasonable chance of identifying many persons with psychiatric or substance use complications. More likely, if patients get past the telephone pre-intake process, they receive an intake assessment or admission. During this time, most programs conduct a more thorough assessment to determine the relative risk the patient brings to the treatment program, both in terms of substance use as well as medical and psychiatric problem severity. The program may use a rational clinical decision-making process to assign the patient to an appropriate level of care. The *ASAM PPC-2R* dimensions I (withdrawal/risk complications), II (biomedical complications), and III (emotional/behavioral/cognitive complications) may be especially useful in this process.

Addiction treatment programs that have evolved to accept patients with co-occurring psychiatric disorders will not deflect or refer those with more stable problems. Instead the focus might be on identifying those with more acute problems. In other words, persons with mood, anxiety, PTSD, or even Axis II or schizophrenic spectrum disorders may be admitted to the program, provided the symptoms are stable. If, however, a person with any of these diagnoses is in an acute state, broadly defined, it may be more likely that this person is not accepted for addiction treatment, even if warranted by level of care considerations.

Factors commonly associated with psychiatric acuity include

- suicidality risk (ideation, plan, intent, behavior)
- homicidality risk
- dangerousness
- agitation
- impulsivity
- capacity for self-regulation and/or self-care

Evaluate Your Program Acceptance Based on Acuity Process

As in assessing disorders, all programs should develop systematic ways to assess these factors. Further, some programs may not make much of a distinction between any of these symptoms when considering their past and present risk. Factors such as "agitation" and "capacity for self-regulation and/or self-care" are often proxies for the level to which a patient can participate in a rigorous schedule of group treatments and meetings, perform responsibilities, and be trusted to live with others in a relatively unsupervised setting. As one program director described, "On weekends we have fifty patients, one staff member, and twenty-three acres. People have got to be able to manage themselves pretty well."

Mental health programs may focus on substance use acuity as well. Is the person actively using substances and what kind? Is the person at risk for withdrawal?

Evaluate an Addiction Treatment Program

In general, an addiction treatment program falls into one of these three categories.

The program

- accepts patients who present with any level of psychiatric symptoms.

- accepts patients who present some psychiatric symptoms but who are diagnosed as stable, not suicidal or homicidal, and who exhibit some level for self-regulation. In the event of crises, these programs tend to rely on outside mental health programs for support.

- accepts patients with all ranges of psychiatric symptoms, including those who may be severe or psychiatrically unstable. These programs provide integrated, comprehensive treatment without having to use a referral system with mental health services.

Evaluate a Mental Health Treatment Program

In general, a mental health treatment program falls into one of these three categories.

The program

- accepts patients who present with any level of acute substance use symptoms.

- accepts patients who present some symptoms of addiction but who are diagnosed as stable, not intoxicated or in withdrawal, and who exhibit some level for self-regulation. In the event of crises, these programs tend to rely on outside addiction treatment programs for support.

- accepts patients with all ranges of addiction symptoms, including those who may be severely addicted, actively using, or at risk for withdrawal. These programs provide integrated, comprehensive treatment without having to use a referral system with addiction treatment services.

Does the person present while intoxicated or is he or she at risk to come to out-patient appointments while under the influence?

Factors commonly associated with substance use acuity include

- intoxication
- withdrawal symptoms or risk
- compulsive or uncontrollable substance use

In assessing your addiction treatment or mental health program, talk with frontline staff, including administrative support personnel who may take the initial referral call. You can also review policy and procedure manuals as well as initial contact and referral forms to determine if acceptance into the program is based on the level of symptoms presented by the individual. In addition, determine if your program is capable of effectively addressing these needs.

Improve Your Program Acceptance Based on Acuity Process
An individual's prior or current level of psychiatric or mental health symptom acuity may affect his or her acceptance into a treatment program.

Programs at the AOS level often base admission decisions on psychiatric history, present diagnosis, or medications. It is often the case that this level program does not have the capacity or staffing to handle an individual with acute mental health symptoms.

Programs at the MHOS level often base admission decisions on substance use history, present diagnoses, or medications. It is often the case that this level program does not have the capacity or staffing to handle an individual with acute substance use symptoms.

To move to the DDC level, an AOS or MHOS program should no longer make acceptance decisions based on the criteria previously listed. Instead, these programs should accept stable individuals regardless of prior hospitalizations, diagnoses, or medications. To move to the DDE level, an AOS or MHOS program must accept and provide treatment to both stable and unstable individuals. This requires having qualified staff members, protocols for patient monitoring and observation, and clear crisis and emergency procedures. Outpatient programs may find this to be easier to achieve than residential or certain inpatient settings.

Program Acceptance Based on Severity
Is program acceptance based on severity and persistence of the psychiatric disability? In addition to acuity, programs may make admission decisions based on

the categories of the disorder in question. AOS programs may feel ill-equipped to assess and/or treat a person with a moderate to severe mental health disorder, even if the patient is relatively stable. In the same way, MHOS programs may feel unprepared to assess and/or treat a patient with a moderate to severe substance use disorder, especially if the patient seems unstable.

The fear is that if these conditions were to deteriorate during treatment, these programs would lack adequate staffing, training, procedures, settings, or support to be able to safely respond. DDC programs are more likely to pay closer attention to the acuity of the problem, and less to the "name" of the diagnosis than AOS and MHOS programs. Much like acuity, however, the severity and persistence classification of the disorder may be based on many things. Most typical are expectations about a given patient's disability, diagnosis, functionality, and "fit" into programmatic expectations.

Severity and persistence of the disorder are often associated with the potential to function within the context of the program. This programmatic expectation may involve fulfilling the responsibilities of the program itself (attending and participating in groups, completing assignments) and also the program milieu (house chores, community living). History of disability, functionality, and fit into programmatic expectations are three ways this issue is often determined. Patient diagnosis is perhaps the most common way. Patients with schizophrenic spectrum disorders, borderline personality disorders, or disorders involving thought disturbances are not accepted into AOS programs and, with careful attention to risk and acuity, sometimes not into a DDC addiction treatment program. Persons with alcohol or drug dependence disorders, or even persons who have alcohol or drug abuse disorders, often are seen as "too severe" to many mental health providers.

Evaluate Your Program Acceptance Based on Severity Process
To learn about your program's approach, interview administrative and clinical staff members who work with referrals and new admissions. Review your clinical protocols and procedures to determine if the program bases services on severity as defined by the diagnosis, persistence, and disability. This serves as an indicator to help determine patients' needs and whether your program is capable of effectively addressing those needs.

Improve Your Program Acceptance Based on Severity Process
Unlike acuity, this dimension pertains to the severity and persistence of the disorder. It is not so much based on the here and now as it is based on the history of

the disorder and the expected course. Rationale for excluding patients based on the type of disorder are sometimes based on policy (certification, licensure, financing) but are oftentimes based on a program's narrative history: "Patients like that don't do well in our program."

AOS programs intending to move to the DDC level will need to accept patients for services who have histories and/or current mental health diagnoses that may be associated with severity and impairment. These diagnostic categories may include mood disorders, anxiety disorders, PTSD, and Axis II disorders, as well as persons with schizophrenia or bipolar disorders. DDC addiction treatment programs will often accept persons who are stable with a non-severe mental illness (often known as a person from quadrant III). See information on the quadrant model of co-occurring disorders in SAMHSA's *Report to Congress on the Prevention and Treatment of Co-occurring Substance Abuse Disorders and Mental Disorders,* 2002. A link to this report is provided on the CD-ROM that accompanies this guidebook. Also see chapter 2 of this guidebook for more information on the quadrant model.

Evaluate an Addiction Treatment Program

*In general, an addiction treatment program's **acceptance based on severity** falls into one of three categories.*

The program accepts patients who

- have no current, or a very limited history of, functional impairment (person's capacity to manage relationships, job, finances, and social interactions) as a result of a psychiatric disorder.

- have mild to moderate histories of functional impairment as a result of a psychiatric disorder. In this case, there may be some substantial history of recurrence of the psychiatric disorder, and/or there has been evidence of continued impairment in at least one functional area (relationships, job, finances, and social interactions). People with Axis I mood disorders, anxiety disorders, PTSD, or Axis II disorders might be more typically served by this program.

- have chronic and potentially lifelong functional impairment as a result of a psychiatric disorder, including persons with severe and persistent mental illnesses. In this case, there may be a significant history of multiple recurrences of the mental health disorder, and/or there has been evidence of continued impairment in several functional areas (relationships, job, finances, and social interactions). Persons with thought disorders (such as schizophrenia and schizoaffective disorder) or severe mood disorders (such as bipolar disorder or major depression) may be served by this program.

Programs clearly operating at the DDC level will also routinely accept persons with less severe bipolar disorder but far less often persons with schizophrenic spectrum disorders, even with current stable clinical status.

DDC addiction treatment programs who seek to move to the DDE level on program acceptance will need to extend their program acceptance to patients in both quadrant III (mood, anxiety, PTSD, less severe Axis II disorders) and quadrant IV (schizophrenia, bipolar disorder, schizoaffective disorder) on a more routine basis. These liberal program acceptance policies are based on clinical appropriateness and are not just an unrealistic willingness to accept all patients at admission. DDE programs must have a clear capacity to effectively treat persons at high levels of severity and acuity.

MHOS programs intending to move to the DDC level will need to accept patients for services who have histories and/or current substance use diagnoses that may be associated with severity and impairment. DDC mental health programs will often accept persons who are stable with a low to moderate level of substance use disorder. To move to the DDE level, mental health programs will need to be able to manage patients with substance use dependence-level disorders.

Research describing this distinction and the manner in which programs vary can be found at http://dms.dartmouth.edu/prc/dual/atsr.

Evaluate a Mental Health Treatment Program

*In general, a mental health treatment program's **acceptance based on severity** falls into one of three categories.*

The program provides care to patients who either

- have no history, or a very limited history of, functional impairment (person's capacity to manage relationships, job, finances, and social interactions) as a result of a substance use disorder.

- have mild to moderate histories of functional impairment as a result of a substance use disorder. In this case, there may be some substantial history of recurrence of the substance use disorder, and/or there has been evidence of continued impairment in at least one functional area (relationships, job, finances, and social interactions).

- have chronic and potentially lifelong functional impairment as a result of a substance use disorder, including persons with severe and persistent addiction. In this case, there may be a significant history of multiple recurrences of the addiction, and/or there has been evidence of continued impairment in several functional areas (relationships, job, finances, and social interactions).

Assessment of Patient Motivation and Preference

Does your program use a stage-wise assessment to identify a patient's motivation to change? In the past, addiction treatment providers assessed patient motivation based on actions not words. A patient was typically categorized as "ready" or "not ready." The latter category often was understood to mean that the patient had yet to hit bottom or, more often, that the patient was suffering from denial—the common reality distortion associated with addiction. Although denial may have a scientific basis in the neurological changes associated with chronic substance use, as well as the correlate cognitive impairment, the above terminology is now being replaced by the stages of change model. Based on the research of James Prochaska and Carlo DiClemente, and translated therapeutically into motivational interviewing by William Miller and Stephen Rollnick, an extensive amount of literature now exists describing this model and its application.

This stage-wise model categorizes each patient into one of four stages (precontemplation, contemplation, preparation and action, and maintenance) that describes the patient's attitudes toward change. This model of behavioral change is well researched with addictive behavior, and its vernacular has been adopted by many community addiction and mental health providers. Two therapeutic models grew out of the stages of change theory: motivational interviewing (MI) and motivational enhancement therapy (MET), which are approaches that community addiction treatment providers can learn and implement easily.

Matching treatment to the patient's attitude toward change (his or her stage in the behavioral change model) is considered a preferred practice. For example, relapse prevention approaches for a patient at the precontemplation stage would likely be an ineffective mismatch, as would be motivational enhancement therapy for a patient who had already recognized his or her problem and was taking steps to heal. For these reasons, assessing motivation is generally seen as an important aspect of assessing readiness for change among persons with substance use disorders.

The model has some inherent problems, however, in that it focuses primarily on cognition and not behavior. Problems in defining the time frame for motivational cognitions (one week, one month, or now?) may alter the rating of the patient's stage. Variable motivations for different substances (e.g., the patient may want to stop using cocaine, but doesn't see alcohol as a problem) also make for measurement challenges.

The Dartmouth group has developed a behavioral measure of substance use treatment, which is aligned with the stages of change model. This Stage of

Treatment Rating Scale is completed by clinicians and is meant to describe the therapeutic behavior (and task) the patient is demonstrating. The four stages go from engagement to persuasion to active treatment to relapse prevention.

It's important to match the stages of change and stages of treatment models.

FIGURE 2

Stages of Change and Stages of Treatment Models

STAGE OF CHANGE	STAGE OF TREATMENT
Precontemplation	Engagement
Contemplation	Persuasion
Action	Active treatment
Maintenance	Relapse prevention

This combination of emphasis on cognition and behavior may be more appropriate when assessing people with co-occurring disorders in clinical settings.

Systematically assessing motivation to address and treat substance use problems is recommended for all providers. An evolving limitation to these models is the lack of attention to differential motivation to address co-occurring psychiatric and substance use problems. Accordingly, new research is seeking to examine the effect of differential patient motivation to address either or both the substance use and psychiatric problem.

For example, Jim suffers from bipolar disorder and alcohol dependence. Jim is very motivated (action stage) to manage his bipolar disorder. He is willing to take medication, meet regularly with his psychiatrist, and participate in weekly group therapy with a clinical social worker (active treatment). But Jim has no interest in dealing with his alcohol use and believes that it is entirely under his willful control.

In contrast, Sam also suffers from bipolar disorder and alcohol dependence. Recently Sam lost his driver's license and got a divorce due to his alcohol use. Sam recognizes that many of his problems stem from alcohol use, including mood swings and financial problems. Although Sam's doctor diagnosed him with bipolar disorder, Sam believes his problem is with alcohol and that once he gets clean and sober, his mood will right itself.

It's important to note that while both Sam and Jim have co-occurring disorders, each is at a different stage of acceptance. While Jim accepts his mental health diagnosis, he is not convinced that he has a substance use problem and he is not interested in addiction treatment.

Sam is decidedly more motivated to stop drinking and seek addiction treatment, but does not accept the diagnosis of his mental health disorder, and is not open to treatment for the disorder.

Assess a Patient's Stage of Motivation for Both Substance Use and Mental Health Disorders

Assessing motivation at both cognitive and behavioral levels for both substance use and mental health problems is seen as critical in the assessment phase of clinical practice. One approach to do this is to have the clinician rate each disorder listed (e.g., on an assessment form or diagnostic summary list) with a corresponding stage-wise rating.

Another approach is using the Stage of Motivation and Treatment Readiness for Co-occurring Disorders (SOMTR-COD) scale, which asks clinicians to provide global ratings on both substance use and mental health problems and to reassess patient motivation over the course of treatment. A reproducible copy of this scale is

---

There are several available measures to assess the stage of motivation. Two established self-report measures that are available online and assess motivation for substance use change within a cognitive framework are

- University of Rhode Island Change Assessment (URICA): www.uri.edu/research

- Stages of Change Readiness and Treatment Eagerness Scale (SOCRATES): http://casaa.unm.edu/inst/SOCRATESv8.pdf

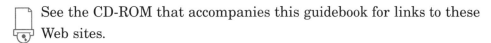 See the CD-ROM that accompanies this guidebook for links to these Web sites.

A clinician-completed measure is also available to assess treatment behavior in terms along a continuum of observable motivation:

- Substance Abuse Treatment Scale (SATS): http://dms.dartmouth.edu/prc/instruments/WebSATS.pdf

---

on the CD-ROM included with this guidebook. Curriculum ❶ *Screening and Assessment* also contains a copy of the scale.

FIGURE 3

Stage-Wise Model of Readiness for Change Matched to Intervention Goals and Treatment Strategies

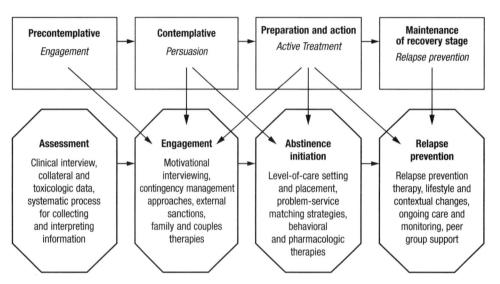

From McGovern, M. P., Wrisley, B. R., & Drake, R. E. (2005). Special section on relapse prevention: Relapse of substance use disorder and its prevention among persons with co-occurring disorders. *Psychiatric Services, 56,* 1270–1273.

Evaluate Your Assessment of Patient Motivation and Preference

Program performance on this benchmark can be determined via interviews and reviews of medical records to determine if the program clinician assesses an individual's readiness for change for substance use and psychiatric disorders when the clinician develops a plan for services. A patient's readiness for change can greatly affect the success of treatment and/or recovery. Taking this aspect into consideration makes for a more comprehensive, strategic, and efficient approach to determining what level of service is most appropriate.

Improve Your Assessment of Patient Motivation and Preference

Assessing the individual's motivation and readiness for change is essential to comprehensive treatment planning. Numerous models exist to define and classify each stage. Motivational interviewing (MI) and motivational enhancement therapies (MET) are arguably evidence-based practices that depend on a careful assessment of patient motivation. One common factor between the various approaches is that individuals can be classified as "ready" or "not ready."

For AOS and MHOS programs to move to the DDC level, they need to identify and note a patient's level of motivational change.

To move to the DDE level, a program must incorporate an assessment of the level of motivation for change, instead of simply identifying the stage. This assessment can include incorporation of the well-established measures (URICA, SOCRATES, SATS) or training staff to develop ratings on the *ASAM PPC-2R* Treatment Acceptance/Resistance dimension (dimension IV). DDE programs also consistently and systematically record this information in patient medical records. Other DDE programs use global ratings of cognitive and treatment behavior readiness for each problem identified in an assessment or diagnostic summary.

AOS or MHOS programs do not routinely assess patient motivation in a stage-based format. DDC programs routinely assess either a substance use or mental health motivation in a stage-based format, and DDE programs assess motivation for both substance use and mental health problems in a stage-based, systematic format.

Simple patient self-report questionnaires can be implemented to help gauge an individual's perception of their own readiness to accept treatment for substance use or mental health disorders. A sample questionnaire that can be customized for your use is included on the CD-ROM that accompanies this guidebook.

Evaluate an Addiction or Mental Health Treatment Program

In general, AOS and MHOS programs fall into one of four categories.

The program

- does not assess an individual's readiness for change.

- occasionally (less than 80 percent of the time) assesses readiness for change in individuals, but the process that is used is informal and clinician-driven.

- includes an assessment of readiness for change within another assessment tool that is already used; this information is documented regularly (at least 80 percent of the time) and focuses on either substance use or mental health motivations.

- assesses readiness for change using a standardized assessment tool for this specific purpose and results are documented regularly, and focuses on both substance use and mental health motivations. If the individual is at different stages for different disorders, this information is documented and measured.

Duplicating this page is illegal. Do not copy this material without written permission from the publisher.

67

FIGURE 4

Simple Patient Self-Report Questionnaire

On a 10-point scale, how much do you want to change your substance use now?

    Not at all   1 -------------------------------- 10   Totally

On a 10-point scale, how sure are you that you will be able to make this change?

    Not at all   1 -------------------------------- 10   Totally

On a 10-point scale, how much do you want to change your mental health problem?

    Not at all   1 -------------------------------- 10   Totally

On a 10-point scale, how sure are you that you will be able to make this change?

    Not at all   1 -------------------------------- 10   Totally

Variants of the stages of change model include an emphasis on the patient who wants to change (or not) and who wants help in doing so (or not). The stages of change model has been criticized for its cognitive emphasis, so other approaches include more of a behavioral focus to identify the steps a patient is willing to take for treatment and the patient's behavioral demonstrations of change.

• • •

Clinical Practice: Evaluating Treatment Approaches

Chapter 6 established the fact that clinical practice is the most central issue that affects an organization's capacity to offer integrated treatment for people with co-occurring disorders. Clinical practice is affected by assessment, treatment, and continuity of care. Chapter 6 evaluated assessment as an important part

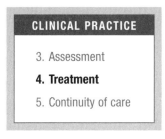

CLINICAL PRACTICE

3. Assessment
4. Treatment
5. Continuity of care

of clinical practice. This chapter offers specific instructions on how you can evaluate and improve the treatment process of your clinical practice. Chapter 8 will complete the analysis of clinical practice by explaining the importance of continuity of care in treating people with co-occurring disorders.

Treatment constitutes the largest number of benchmarks of all the seven dimensions of the DDCAT index. Treatment of co-occurring disorders fundamentally rests on the assumption demonstrated by the early work of McLellan et al. on problem-service matching: Patient outcomes improve when mental health and substance use problems are treated (McLellan, Lewis, O'Brien, & Kleber, 2000).

In the sections that follow, the ten treatment practice benchmarks are defined in detail, and examples of programs that are operating at DDC and DDE levels are given. Suggestions for how a program may consider enhancing its performance on each benchmark are also noted. The ten benchmarks define specific practices that can be implemented by an addiction treatment or mental health treatment program. Some may require certain type of personnel (e.g., a prescriber for medication), but most do not.

Understanding Your Program's Treatment Practices

The ten treatment benchmarks focus very specifically on a program's approach to practice. As with the assessment benchmarks discussed in the previous chapter, the treatment benchmarks value a consistent and systematic approach to address a patient's symptoms of mental health and/or substance use disorders. The more protocol-driven (versus individual clinician-driven) a program's treatment practice is, the better. This is why several of the ten benchmarks focus on documenting the consistency of treatment in medical records or patient charts. Other benchmarks examine the implementation of certain practices: medications, psychosocial treatments, stage-wise treatments, involvement of family/significant others in treatment, and peer recovery supports.

TREATMENT PRACTICE BENCHMARKS

Treatment practice refers to ten specific benchmarks that should be evaluated in this order:

1. Treatment plan focus
2. Monitoring co-occurring disorders during treatment
3. Standard procedures for psychiatric and substance-related emergencies and crises
4. Stage-wise treatment
5. Medication management
6. Specialized psychosocial interventions
7. Patient education
8. Family education
9. Specialized interventions for peer support
10. Access to peer recovery role models

Many health care providers are under the impression that the *only* treatment approach for psychiatric problems is medication. In fact, the psychosocial treatments (such as CBT) for the most common disorders (mood, anxiety, PTSD, and social phobia) surpass medications in effectiveness. Most other psychiatric disorders (e.g., bipolar disorder, depression, and anxiety disorders) have FDA-approved medications indicated for them; however, patient outcomes are improved substantially when medications are combined with psychotherapies. Other mental health disorders, such as Axis II disorders, have fewer effective medication options. The belief that only medications can be used to treat co-occurring psychiatric disorders is a myth.

Treatment Plan Focus

In your program, do treatment or recovery plans address both psychiatric and substance-related disorders? Most funding authorities and payers of services require a treatment plan document. This plan typically lists a problem or goal, an objective (a bite-size chunk of a problem that is often more observable), an intervention, a person responsible for delivering the intervention, and a target date. Many programs or clinicians ask patients to review these plans, and for this reason the road map to their care is transparent and collaborative. This is an excellent, often underutilized, pratice.

Addiction treatment services vary considerably. Many addiction treatment programs, typically AOS programs, attempt to treat only the substance use disorder. Other addiction treatment programs focus on treating the substance use disorder, but see psychiatric disorders as complications to recovery, so as with any other complication (e.g., medical, legal, social), they try to identify the mental health disorder and then offer treatment or refer the patient to outside treatment. In the same way, many mental health programs treat only the psychiatric disorder. Some mental health programs focus on the psychiatric disorder, but see substance use disorders as a complication to recovery. These programs may assess and identify a substance use disorder and may refer the patient to outside addiction treatment services. Other addiction treatment or mental health treatment programs see substance use and psychiatric problems as being closely intertwined, so they provide treatment for both.

For AOS programs, the treatment plan may focus entirely on substance use and substance-related issues. In decades past, addiction programs might list "alcoholism" as the problem and list a short-term treatment objective. The primary counselor's name would be noted as the key person responsible, and the target date would be "by discharge."

Most AOS programs have evolved to become more specific and precise in the identification of goals (e.g., reduce symptoms of alcohol dependence) and objectives (provide patient education, meet with the patient and his or her family to build recovery support, develop relapse prevention skills, solidify motivation, and so on). Typically, a clinician meets with a team of responsible individuals, including the patient, to develop these goals and objectives. Nonetheless, AOS programs do not often list a psychiatric problem on the treatment plan, even if the disorder was identified during the assessment process.

Most MHOS programs are similar to AOS programs in that they are relatively specific and precise in the identification of goals (e.g., reduce symptoms of a mental health disorder) and objectives (provide patient education, meet with the patient and his or her family to build recovery support, develop life skills, solidify motivation, and so on). Clinicians in these programs often utilize a team of responsible individuals, along with the patient, to develop these goals and objectives. Nonetheless, MHOS programs do not often list a substance use problem on the treatment plan, even if a significant substance use disorder was identified during the assessment process.

The DDC-level addiction treatment or mental health program often retains a closer link in sequence between the clinical practice of assessment and treatment. A co-occurring disorder, once identified during assessment, does find its way onto the treatment plan. Some intentions to address it and to monitor it are outlined. These may include referrals to a mental health or addiction treatment provider off-site, or a consulting provider on-site. Interventions may involve an adaptation of group and/or individual treatments so that the patient at least receives some ongoing support for the co-occurring condition.

The DDE-level addiction treatment or mental health program lists both the substance use problem and the mental health problem, and the order could be interchangeable, since both are clearly a primary focus.

Evaluate Your Treatment Plan Focus

To understand your program's approach, a simple place to start is to examine records of treatment and recovery plans. Is there a format clinicians use to record both disorders and target treatments accordingly? If there is a format that could capture both disorders on a plan, how is this format used? Even the most sophisticated formats may still list alcoholism as the problem, and steps one, two, and three as the short-term goals. In reviewing how the forms are completed, do you

---

Evaluate an Addiction Treatment Program

In general, the focus of an addiction treatment program fits into one of these five categories.

The treatment or recovery plan focus is on

- substance use disorders only.

- substance use disorders primarily, with occasional focus on psychiatric disorders. This can be due to clinician preferences and competencies, time constraints, or resources.

- both substance use and psychiatric disorders; however, recovery planning tends to focus on substance use disorders with brief, nonspecific references to mental health concerns.

- both substance use and psychiatric disorders equally and in detail; however, not all recovery plans go into equal levels of detail about both.

- both substance use and psychiatric disorders equally, in specific detail, and with consistency; this is indicated by clear and measurable objectives for both substance use and mental health disorders.

---

notice consistency from clinician to clinician, or is there a wide variation in how the treatment and recovery plans are dealt with?

At this juncture it's important to acknowledge that many will view the focus on this benchmark (i.e., documentation in treatment plans) as superficial, mechanical, and bureaucratic. Many clinicians will divulge that they write as little as possible on the record, ostensibly either to protect the patient or so that they can focus on the true art of actually talking with patients. Many of the most talented clinicians are notorious for being the worst record keepers, and perhaps the best record keeper can be the most ineffective clinician. How to rectify these issues is beyond the scope of this guidebook; yet the record can be beneficial because it provides some measure of consistency in the clinical process. If the treatment or recovery plan is to reflect an explicit contractual document between provider and patient, it should also more closely correspond to reality.

In addition, some experts believe that having a format to capture and guide these sorts of clinical processes can help train new clinicians more quickly (since every note is not a blank white page) by fostering a clinical discipline and therapeutic focus. Other experts point to the fact that by creating a series of steps in a medical record, electronic or otherwise, a clinical supervisor can support the implementation of a given practice. Programs should consider using a consistent format in a treatment or recovery plan to help support clinicians in tuning in to both substance use and psychiatric problems. This format should be built to

Evaluate a Mental Health Treatment Program

In general, the focus of a mental health program fits into one of these five categories.

The treatment or recovery plan focus is on

- psychiatric disorders only.

- psychiatric disorders primarily, with occasional focus on substance use disorders. This can be due to clinician preferences and competencies, time constraints, or resources.

- both substance use and psychiatric disorders; however, recovery planning tends to focus on psychiatric disorders with brief, nonspecific references to mental health concerns.

- both substance use and psychiatric disorders equally and in detail; however, not all recovery plans go into equal levels of detail about both.

- both substance use and psychiatric disorders equally, in specific detail, and with consistency; this is indicated by clear and measurable objectives for both substance use and mental health disorders.

accommodate both substance use and mental health disorders and clinician and patient perspectives.

Improve Your Treatment Plan Focus

Treatment planning can begin after the program staff assesses and interacts with the patient. Typically the patient and program staff work together to set goals using a shared decision-making process. The best example of this is the research on therapeutic alliance in psychotherapy.

For an AOS program to move to the DDC level, the program must begin to not only screen, assess, diagnose, and identify psychiatric disorders, but must also develop a treatment plan that targets and monitors the identified problems. Similarly, in order for an MHOS program to move to the DDC level, the program must begin to not only screen, assess, diagnose, and identify substance use disorders, but must also develop a treatment plan that targets and monitors the identified problems.

For any program to move to the DDE level, the treatment for substance use and psychiatric disorders should be equal and documented, generally managed, and conducted "in house." Objectives for treatment should be specific and may include interventions in relation to medications and psychosocial treatments.

Monitoring Co-occurring Disorders during Treatment

Does your program assess and monitor interactive courses of both disorders? Since substance use and psychiatric disorders are interrelated and dynamic, it is important to review the patient's progress, or lack thereof, on each disorder. For instance, John is a patient who has recently been admitted into an addiction treatment center for alcoholism. John scored high on an initial screening measure for depression. John also has a positive family history for mood disorders. The addiction treatment clinician that screened John found that he reported severe symptoms of depression that predated the onset of his alcohol use problem. John also reported depressive symptoms during times of abstinence from alcohol. During the first two weeks of addiction treatment, John's mood symptoms improved significantly. This may mean that John is no longer suffering from symptoms of depression, but it probably does not mean that he no longer suffers from a mood disorder. John's depressive symptoms must be monitored over the next two weeks. One would hope that he will continue to report a positive mood. In people being treated for substance use disorders, mood and anxiety symptoms often return to normal within the first month of addiction treatment. Patients' symptoms may change, sometimes quickly. The key practice in treatment is the capacity to monitor these changes, to record the observations systematically (by providing a format for clinicians), and to adjust the treatment if needed.

Evaluate Your Monitoring of Co-occurring Disorders during Treatment

To learn about this treatment benchmark in your program, you will need to review your program's medical records and formats and processes and procedures for monitoring co-occurring symptoms and disorders. Determine if both disorders, as well as the interactive course of the disorders, is continually assessed and monitored. (See the box at the bottom of this page and on page 76 to evaluate an addiction or mental health treatment program.)

Improve Your Monitoring of Co-occurring Disorders during Treatment

Abstinence from alcohol and other drugs will affect a patient's psychiatric symptoms. Assessing, monitoring, and documenting a patient's current and continuing abstinence plays a vital role in the development of a comprehensive treatment plan.

AOS programs may list the chronologies of disorders, though usually not in a standardized or consistent fashion. Treatment, therefore, does not rely on the possibility of a change in level of psychiatric symptoms with abstinence.

To move to the DDC level, AOS programs should consistently record the chronologies of all disorders and should monitor for psychiatric symptom or substance use changes early on in the patient's treatment. DDC programs also help prepare the patient for the possibility that psychiatric symptoms may return even if he or she remains abstinent from alcohol and other drugs. If the patient's

---

Evaluate an Addiction Treatment Program

In general, an addiction treatment program will fall into one of these five categories.

The monitoring of patient symptoms during treatment will

- focus on substance use disorders only.
- irregularly focus on co-occurring psychiatric disorders, varying by clinician.
- regularly focus on co-occurring psychiatric disorders in a basic way, usually by including a generic description of the disorder in the patient's medical record.
- regularly focus on co-occurring psychiatric disorders in a basic way. In some instances there is a more systematic and equally in-depth focus on both mental health and substance use disorders, although this is done on an irregular basis.
- regularly focus on co-occurring psychiatric disorders in a detailed, systematic, and in-depth way. This continued monitoring is documented in a standardized fashion within the record.

---

psychiatric symptoms do return, the DDC program documents this information. To move to the DDE level, changes in mental health and addiction symptoms are more regularly monitored and recorded by using more in-depth medical records or timeline follow-back (TLFB) calendars.

Similarly, MHOS programs may also list the chronologies of disorders, though usually not in a standardized or consistent fashion. Treatment, therefore, does not rely on the possibility of a change in level of substance use symptoms as mental health treatment progresses. To move to the DDC level, MHOS programs should more consistently record the chronologies of all disorders and should monitor for changes in substance use symptoms early on in the individual's treatment. DDC programs also help prepare individuals for the possibility that substance use symptoms may return even after mental health symptoms improve. If this does occur, the DDC program documents this information. To move to the DDE level, these changes in symptoms are more regularly monitored and recorded by using more in-depth medical records or TLFB calendars.

Standard Procedures for Psychiatric and Substance-Related Emergencies and Crises

Are there standard procedures for psychiatric and substance-related emergencies and crisis management?

As a program expands the portal within which patients with co-occurring disorders can enter, the need to develop emergency protocols will arise. Many

---

Evaluate a Mental Health Treatment Program

In general, a mental health treatment program will fall into one of these five categories.

The monitoring of patient symptoms during treatment will

- focus on psychiatric disorders only.
- irregularly focus on co-occurring substance use disorders, varying by clinician.
- regularly focus on co-occurring substance use disorders in a basic way, usually by including a generic description of the disorder in the patient's medical record.
- regularly focus on co-occurring substance use disorders in a basic way. In some instances there is a more systematic and equally in-depth focus on both mental health and substance use disorders, although this is done on an irregular basis.
- regularly focus on co-occurring substance use disorders in a detailed, systematic, and in-depth way. This continued monitoring is documented in a standardized fashion within the record.

---

programs have only the "9-1-1" emergency response telephone number when the rare situation occurs (once every several years) that requires additional help. Other programs expect emergencies and crises as more commonplace and perhaps as associated with the course of certain psychiatric or substance use disorders.

An outpatient treatment program in the Midwest made concerted efforts to expand services to persons with co-occurring disorders. The staff hired new counselors, developed treatment groups, and used a grant from United Way to hire a case manager. They began accepting referrals directly from the local state hospital. Many of these patients were not stable in recovery from either substance use or psychiatric disorders. As such, the need to transport patients to the local hospital emergency service or state hospital crisis service increased from once every few years to once or twice per month. The agency's leadership recognized this unanticipated emerging need and developed more specific protocols and charter agreements with the local hospital and state hospital providers.

Evaluate Your Standard Procedures for Psychiatric and Substance-Related Emergencies and Crises

To evaluate your program's guidelines on emergency response, start with a discussion with key clinical staff members and review the program's clinical protocols used in mental health crises. Ask if your program includes standard guidelines or procedures for emergency response, either written or unwritten.

Evaluate an Addiction Treatment Program

*In general, an addiction treatment program's guidelines on **emergency response** fall into one of these four categories.*

The program may

- have no plan, written or unwritten, to deal with mental health emergencies or crises.

- have no written plan for handling emergency situations; however, the staff can verbalize how to handle a crisis beyond calling emergency personnel. The staff has a sense of intervention options as well as how a crisis might affect its institution as a whole.

- have some written guidelines for mental health crises and may have made arrangements with mental health clinics and other providers to assist when called upon. Intervention strategies are also included in these written guidelines.

- have explicit and thoroughly written guidelines that include in-house management of crises. This means that the program is capable of ongoing risk assessment and management of persons with interacting and elevating symptoms.

CLINICAL ADMINISTRATOR'S GUIDEBOOK

Improve Your Standard Procedures for Psychiatric and Substance-Related Emergencies and Crises

Many AOS programs do not have the capacity to accept patients who may have psychiatric emergencies. Similarly, many MHOS programs do not have the capacity to accept patients who may have substance use emergencies. For this reason, these individuals are usually not accepted into any program (whether mental health or addiction treatment) that seeks to keep the number of emergency situations to a minimum.

To move to the DDC level, AOS and MHOS programs must create a more formalized, standard, and documented protocol that the staff can then clearly verbalize. This may include calling upon outside mental health agencies, the nearby hospital, or emergency services. In some instances, DDC programs may be capable of handling the emergency in-house if the staff has been trained in risk management and assessment. DDE programs, due to the nature of individuals who are admitted, expect to deal with emergency situations on a more regular basis. The programs at this level, therefore, have clear, articulated, documented plans as well as the capacity to deal with situations in-house. This, in turn, means there are never issues with referrals or linking to outside agencies.

Evaluate a Mental Health Treatment Program

*In general, a mental health treatment program's guidelines on **emergency response** fall into one of these four categories.*

The program may

- have no plan, written or unwritten, to deal with substance use emergencies or crises.

- have no written plan for handling emergency situations; however, the staff can verbalize how to handle a crisis beyond calling emergency personnel. The staff has a sense of intervention options as well as how a crisis might affect its institution as a whole.

- have some written guidelines for substance use crises and may have made arrangements with addiction treatment clinics and other providers to assist when called upon. Intervention strategies are also included in these written guidelines.

- have explicit and thoroughly written guidelines that include in-house management of crises. This means that the program is capable of ongoing risk assessment and management of persons with interacting and elevating symptoms.

Stage-Wise Treatment

It is clinically important to consider the stage of patient motivation (and treatment behavior) when matching specific interventions. For example, it would not be appropriate to put a patient in the Precontemplation stage for a substance use disorder in an ongoing relapse prevention group. Likewise, it would not be appropriate to put an alcoholic patient at the Maintenance stage in an early-engagement program with education on the basics of addiction, instead of a program that covered long-term relapse prevention.

Different evidence-based practices are indicated for patients at certain stages of motivation to change behavior. Figure 5 shows the stage-wise model of readiness for change. This model does not match treatment approaches to patient readiness for patients who suffer from both substance use and mental health disorders. Instead, this model shows how addiction treatment approaches should match patient readiness. This model is helpful in understanding how different levels of patient motivation correlate to appropriate stages of addiction treatment.

FIGURE 5

Stage-Wise Model of Readiness for Change Matched to Intervention Goals and Treatment Strategies

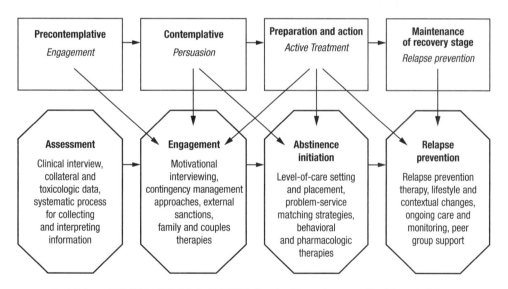

From McGovern, M. P., Wrisley, B. R., & Drake, R. E. (2005). Special section on relapse prevention: Relapse of substance use disorder and its prevention among persons with co-occurring disorders. *Psychiatric Services, 56,* 1270–1273.

Different evidence-based practices are indicated for patients at certain stages of motivation to change behavior. Figure 6 considers both the mental health disorder and the substance use disorder when matching the appropriate treatment approaches to one of four levels of patient readiness to change: precontemplation, contemplation, action, and maintenance. This model is helpful in understanding how different levels of patient motivation correlate to appropriate stages of treatment for both substance use and mental health disorders. The matter of assessing patient motivation is complicated when one considers the differential motivation for mental health issues. This assessment should occur at both cognitive and behavioral levels.

FIGURE 6

Stage, Substance Use Problem, and Mental Health Problem

STAGE	SUBSTANCE USE PROBLEM	MENTAL HEALTH PROBLEM
Precontemplation	Motivational enhancement therapy; contingency management; marital/family therapies	Motivational enhancement therapy; contingency management; marital/family therapies
Contemplation	Patient education	Patient education
Action	Therapeutic environment for stablization; cognitive-behavioral therapy; pharmacotherapy	Therapeutic environment for stablization; cognitive-behavioral therapy; pharmacotherapy
Maintenance	Relapse prevention; ongoing psychotherapy; recovery monitoring; peer recovery support groups	Relapse prevention; ongoing psychotherapy; recovery monitoring; peer recovery support groups

The important practice for the addiction treatment program is to assess a patient's stage of motivation and treatment readiness, perhaps by using the Stage of Motivation and Treatment Readiness for Co-occurring Disorders (SOMTR-COD) assessment form found on the CD-ROM that accompanies this guidebook. The form is also found in curriculum ❶ *Screening and Assessment.* This form is designed to be used for the initial assessment and for updated assessments that occur over time. In the more enhanced programs, clinicians will match treatment methods individually to patients, depending on where the patient is according to the four levels of patient readiness to change: precontemplation, contemplation, action, and maintenance.

A debatable issue is whether to group patients at the same stage of motivation together for treatment. For example, a clinician could organize a therapy group for patients in the precontemplation stage, while organizing a separate therapy group for patients in the maintenance stage. Clinicians, especially those trained in group therapy, have long argued for the benefits of group members who are allowed to confront or influence one another. Conversely, some clinicians have emphasized that conducting segregated treatment groups is challenging. Often the concern is that motivated patients will be negatively influenced just as unmotivated patients will be leveraged forward. This debate is beyond the present scope of this guide; however, a programmatic reality may be that only one group, or one topic group, can be conducted at any one time so that patient differentiation on this dimension is not feasible. The key practice is to have the stage of patient motivation in mind when delivering treatments, regardless of whether a patient is in a group with patients at the same stage of motivation.

Evaluate Your Stage-Wise Treatment

To evaluate the stage-wise treatment approaches within your program, first review your program's protocols for continued assessment and monitoring of the patient's stage of motivation. You must then determine if the stages of change contribute to the development of treatment plans and plans for continued services. Assess whether the treatment plan fits each stage in terms of content, intensity, and use of outside agencies. Ask if there is continued follow-up to monitor the patient's stage as it may change over time. As with other benchmarks, systematic and consistent monitoring is valued over clinician-driven and more inconsistent application of this practice.

Evaluate an Addiction or Mental Health Treatment Program

In general, a program falls into one of these four categories.

The program

- does not monitor motivational stages regularly throughout treatment and therefore does not address this issue during the course of treatment.

- occasionally and informally assesses and documents a patient's stage of motivation throughout the course of treatment, if the individual clinician chooses to do so.

- regularly assesses and documents stages of motivation but these stages are not necessarily incorporated into treatments. This is often due to the fact that the treatment plans are more generic, placing individuals into service tracks as opposed to developing individualized plans.

- regularly assesses and documents stages of motivation throughout treatment and develops and utilizes individualized treatment plans targeting these stages.

Improve Your Stage-Wise Treatment

Information regarding an individual's motivational stages is usually gathered during the assessment process. However, AOS or MHOS programs may not include this component in the assessment tool, and it is then left out of treatment planning.

To move to the DDC level, AOS or MHOS programs must consistently assess and document a patient's motivational stage and incorporate that information into his or her treatment plan.

For example, a residential program in Oregon has operationalized the ASAM dimension IV (treatment acceptance or resistance), which reduces the length of stay based on stage of readiness assessed at two-week intervals. Ratings of precontemplation or contemplation stages result in earlier transitions to an intensive outpatient level of care. This conserves a more expensive resource (residential services) and enables patients at action or maintenance stages more access.

For AOS or MHOS programs to move to the DDE level, information about a patient's stage of motivation should be routinely assessed, documented, and incorporated into ever-evolving, individualized treatment plans. DDE programs also pay particular attention to the concept that a patient may be at a different motivational stage for each disorder or issue. DDE programs may also strive to assess differential motivation to address both substance use and psychiatric problems.

Medication Management

What policies and procedures are in place for medication evaluation, management, monitoring, and adherence? FDA-approved medications are evidence-based treatments for many psychiatric and substance use disorders. The specific medications, their indications, and their risks, are fully described in curriculum ❹ *Medication Management*. The available research suggests that medication treatment for psychiatric patients is the same, whether the patient has only a mental health disorder or has a co-occurring substance use disorder. Research also suggests that patients with mental health disorders can benefit from medications for addiction, such as methadone, buprenorphine, acamprosate, naltrexone, or disulfiram.

For example, a person with unipolar depression may be treated with a selective serotonin reuptake inhibitor (SSRI). For the person with bipolar disorder, a mood stabilizer, such as lithium, is indicated. For anxiety disorders, where several anxiolytics as well as benzodiazepines and tranquilizers have addictive potential, SSRIs are most often indicated. For persons with psychotic spectrum disorders, antipsychotics, and perhaps in particular, atypical antipsychotics are indicated. Of course these psychotropic medications work best if the patient with a substance use disorder is abstinent. The medications do not work effectively if the person is not abstinent. Scientific reviews have found that these medications can have a secondary and profoundly therapeutic effect on substance use (e.g., alcohol dependence). However, there is no evidence that psychotropic medications can cure substance use disorders.

Utilizing psychotropic medications for co-occurring psychiatric disorders and addiction medications for alcohol dependence (such as naltrexone, disulfiram, or acamprosate) or opioid dependence (methadone, LAAM, or buprenorphine) would be considered the best possible implementation of combined evidence-based medication practices for co-occurring disorders. Utilizing medications alone, without psychosocial treatments, will probably prove ineffective. Nonetheless, having good access to medications initially, having the capability to adjust medications once prescribed, and having the prescriber be a key part of the treatment team are all important to your program's ability to treat co-occurring disorders.

Evaluate Your Medication Management
In evaluating performance on this treatment benchmark, you can review your program's medication management policies and procedures as well as your prescriber's role. Ask if your program has documented policies and procedures for

---

Evaluate an Addiction or Mental Health Treatment Program

In general, a program falls into one of these five categories.

The program

- lacks the capacity and resources to manage, monitor, or prescribe medications.

- is unable to prescribe medications or has restrictions on the types of medications that can be managed.

- has access to a prescriber who can prescribe medications for individuals with co-occurring disorders in treatment.

- has a prescriber on staff who can prescribe medications to individuals in treatment with co-occurring disorders and monitor these medications; however, this prescriber is not fully integrated into the treatment team. The prescriber often acts independently and is seen as an adjunctive service provider.

- has a prescriber on staff who is fully integrated into the treatment team and is involved in recovery planning and administrative decisions.

evaluating medication needs, coordinating and managing medication regimens, monitoring for adherence to regimens, and responding to any challenges or difficulties with medication adherence.

On this benchmark, the key measure is patient access to needed medication.

Improve Your Medication Management

A program's ability and capacity to prescribe medications may affect admission decisions. AOS programs do not typically prescribe medications for mental health disorders. At best, an AOS program may have informal, undocumented policies for administering a few psychiatric medications. Similarly, MHOS programs do not typically prescribe anti-addiction medications, such as buprenorphine, naltrexone, or acamprosate, or medications for detoxification. MHOS programs may not be aware of the use of methadone for patients with opiate use disorders.

To move to the DDC level, AOS or MHOS programs may need to increase the number of medications managed, as well as develop clear guidelines for administering and managing these medications. Medications should be kept in a secure, locked storage area and be self-administered but observed. Medications may be brought in by a patient, renewed by an outside prescriber, or offered as a new prescription at your program during treatment. Necessary adjustments to a patient's medications can be made during treatment, and written protocols for assessing and documenting these adjustments should be developed. DDC programs document the use of all medications and each patient's compliance in medication use over time. This is evident in each patient's medical record.

To move to the DDE level, the program must have the capacity to administer pharmacotherapy, to monitor toxicology, and to treat individuals actively using medications for medical or psychiatric problems with abuse liability. These protocols are well developed, and the medication response is consistently well documented in each patient's record.

Consider obtaining curriculum ❹ *Medication Management* to improve your services on the medication management benchmark.

Specialized Psychosocial Interventions

Psychosocial treatments such as psychotherapy, counseling, and patient education are the most common vehicles for services in addiction treatment. Most, if not all, addiction treatment programs offer psychosocial services; this includes addiction treatment programs that rely primarily on medication-assisted recovery such as methadone or buprenorphine. Evidence-based psychosocial treatments for addiction are numerous, but most fit into one of these four therapy categories: cognitive and behavioral approach, motivational approaches, family systems, and support groups. Most psychosocial treatments for mental health conditions can also be placed into these categories, with the primary treatment falling into the category of cognitive and behavioral psychology, more so than motivational approaches and recovery group supports.

Generally, these treatments involve a component of patient education. They also include a functional analysis of the antecedents, behaviors, and consequences of the target behavior (e.g., smoking cannabis, panic attack). Psychosocial treatments also involve monitoring behavior, establishing coping alternatives, working to decrease anxiety by increasing exposure to feared stimuli, utilizing reinforcement contingencies, and working to increase a sense of self-efficacy. Improvements in relationships, communication, peer support, and alternative replacement activities are also common results of effective treatment.

Blending together these common elements from addiction treatment and psychiatric treatment is a relatively straightforward process that many practitioners have already established in their programs and offices. Some practitioners have taken handouts and materials from addiction and mental health treatment manuals, photocopied them, and used them in an organized manner with patients who suffer with both a substance use and mental health disorder. Other practitioners have used more specific addiction treatment manuals (e.g., MET or MI) and have modified them informally to fit with patients in group sessions.

Treatment models, each with some research-based evidence accrued or accruing, have been specifically developed for persons with co-occurring substance use and psychiatric disorders. Figure 7 describes the appropriate treatment approach for patients with specific combinations of substance use and psychiatric disorders.

Clinicians can use the clinician's guide from curriculum ❷ *Integrating Combined Therapies* and from curriculum ❸ *Cognitive-Behavioral Therapy* in the Co-occcurring Disorders Program to improve their specialized interventions. These two clinician's guides provide specialized interventions for psychiatric problems common in people suffering from substance use disorders. Please also utilize the resources available at the end of this guidebook for other methods to enhance your treatment services.

FIGURE 7

Psychiatric Disorder, Substance Use Disorder, and Treatment Approach

PSYCHIATRIC DISORDER	SUBSTANCE USE DISORDER	TREATMENT APPROACH
Depression/dysthymia	Alcohol dependence	CBT (Brown & Ramsey, 2000)
Bipolar disorder	Alcohol and/or drug dependence	CBT (Weiss et al., 2007)
Social phobia	Alcohol dependence	CBT (Randall, Thomas, & Thevos, 2001)
PTSD	Cocaine dependence	CBT (Brady, Dansky, Back, Foa, & Carroll, 2001)
	Alcohol and/or drug dependence	Seeking safety (Najavits, in press; Hein, Cohen, Miele, Litt, & Capstick, 2004)
	Alcohol and/or drug dependence	CBT (McGovern, Alterman, Drake, & Dauten, 2008)

Using Psychosocial Interventions

Most addiction treatment providers offer psychosocial treatments in residential, intensive outpatient, and outpatient programs over the course of multiple hours of services. Residential programs may offer up to forty or more hours per week of psychosocial services in the form of groups, meetings, and individual sessions. Intensive outpatient programs offer a minimum of twelve hours per week of services, and outpatient programs may offer as few as one hour per week and as many as eleven hours per week. This means that there are plenty of available hours to integrate psychosocial services for patients with co-occurring psychiatric disorders— especially since at least 50 percent of addiction treatment program patients will have these disorders.

Many addiction treatment programs offer only addiction-focused psychosocial interventions with some being evidence-based, some being idiosyncratic, and others being more traditional. Other addiction programs offer some services that begin to address some co-occurring psychiatric disorder issues. These generic services can be individual sessions where psychiatric disorders are addressed along with a variety of other concerns. They may also be addressed in the context of groups that focus on feelings, anger management, affect management, or communication skills. Many addiction treatment groups of this nature introduce the fact that many members will have co-occurring disorders and the group will help them manage the disorders through increased awareness (this may or may not include education about the psychiatric disorder) and some new coping skills.

Some addiction and mental health providers have attempted to adopt specific practices targeting specific disorders with manual-guided, evidence-based treatments. Since some of these practices were developed for certain populations (e.g., women) and settings (e.g., long-term outpatient programs), providers have been forced to adapt them to their unique settings and patient populations. Nonetheless, this is a sincere effort to provide psychosocial treatment services in an integrated, enhanced fashion.

Evaluate Your Specialized Psychosocial Interventions

To investigate a program's offering of specialized psychosocial interventions for psychiatric disorders, review the program's interventions, practices, recovery plans, and progress notes to determine if they target both mental health and substance use disorders. In addition, assess whether interventions are integrated into treatment and if they are generically applied to programs. These interventions might include stress management, relaxation training, anger management, coping skills, assertiveness training, and problem solving. More advanced mental health interventions include brief motivational or cognitive-behavioral therapies that target specific disorders such as PTSD, depression, anxiety disorders, and Axis II disorders.

Note that this benchmark focuses specifically on psychosocial or behavioral interventions for persons with co-occurring disorders in both addiction and

---

Evaluate an Addiction Treatment Program

In general, a program falls into one of these five categories.

The program

- does not incorporate specialized psychosocial interventions to specifically address mental health concerns, symptoms, or disorders.

- irregularly provides generic interventions for psychiatric concerns, based on individual clinicians.

- routinely incorporates generic, broadly applicable mental health interventions for individuals with co-occurring disorders.

- routinely incorporates generic, broadly applicable mental health interventions for individuals with co-occurring disorders and, with some regularity, offers more individualized interventions for psychiatric disorders.

- routinely provides targeted mental health interventions that are individualized to the disorder. These mental health interventions are comprised of more generic, broadly applicable services, as well as more individualized and skilled interventions that target specific psychiatric disorders.

---

mental health treatment settings. Medications are frequently viewed to be the primary treatment option for psychiatric conditions in addiction settings; however, psychosocial/behavioral interventions should also be an integral component of treatment, as they tend to have longer-lasting affects.

Improve Your Specialized Psychosocial Interventions

Psychosocial interventions should be administered by a trained clinician with experience in therapies for co-occurring disorders or cognitive-behavioral therapy. At this time, there are not many evidence-based treatments, though many are in the development and testing stages. SAMHSA has been making some strides in creating a National Registry of Evidence-based Programs and Practices (NREPP). This effort is in its early stages and far from the level of detail, protocol, and sophistication needed for a comparison with the FDA-approval process used for pharmacological agents. But studies with PTSD (Hein et al., 2004), depression (Brown & Ramsey, 2001), social phobia (Randall et al., 2001) and other diagnostically heterogeneous groups (McEvoy & Nathan, 2007) have supported CBT as a generically effective treatment.

Evaluate a Mental Health Treatment Program

In general, a program falls into one of these five categories.

The program

- does not incorporate specialized psychosocial interventions to specifically address substance use concerns, symptoms, or disorders.

- irregularly provides generic interventions for substance use concerns, based on individual clinicians.

- routinely incorporates generic, broadly applicable substance use interventions for individuals with co-occurring disorders.

- routinely incorporates generic, broadly applicable substance use interventions for individuals with co-occurring disorders and, with some regularity, offers more individualized interventions for substance use disorders.

- routinely provides targeted substance use interventions that are individualized to the disorder. These substance use interventions are comprised of more generic, broadly applicable services, as well as more individualized and skilled interventions that target specific substance use disorders.

Evidence-Based Addiction Treatment Manuals

These addiction treatments can be adapted for use with persons with co-occurring disorders. Visit the CD-ROM ⬚ included with this guidebook for links to these manuals.

NIDA Therapy Manuals for Cocaine Addiction: www.nida.nih.gov/ DrugPages/Treatment.html

1. *A Cognitive-Behavioral Approach: Treating Cocaine Addiction*

2. *A Community Reinforcement Approach: Treating Cocaine Addiction*

3. *An Individual Drug Counseling Approach to Treat Cocaine Addiction: The Collaborative Cocaine Treatment Study Model*

4. *Drug Counseling for Cocaine Addiction: The Collaborative Cocaine Treatment Study Model*

NIAAA Therapy Manuals: http://www.niaaa.nih.gov/

1. *Twelve Step Facilitation Therapy Manual*

2. *Motivational Enhancement Therapy Manual*

3. *Cognitive-Behavioral Coping Skills Therapy Manual*

COMBINE Monograph Series

1. *Combined Behavioral Intervention Manual: A Clinical Research Guide for Therapists Treating People with Alcohol Abuse and Dependence*

SAMHSA Cannabis Youth Treatment Series: http://ncadi.samhsa.gov/

1. *Motivational Enhancement Therapy and Cognitive Behavioral Therapy for Adolescent Cannabis Users: 5 Sessions*

2. *The Motivational Enhancement Therapy and Cognitive Behavioral Therapy Supplement: 7 Sessions of Cognitive Behavioral Therapy for Adolescent Cannabis Users*

3. *Family Support Network Therapy for Adolescent Cannabis Users*

4. *The Adolescent Community Reinforcement Approach for Adolescent Cannabis Users*

5. *Multidimensional Family Therapy for Adolescent Cannabis Users*

SAMHSA Specialized Manuals: www.kap.samhsa.gov

1. *Therapeutic Community Curriculum*

2. Matrix manuals

3. *Anger Management for Substance Abuse and Mental Health Clients: A Cognitive Behavioral Therapy Manual*

Duplicating this page is illegal. Do not copy this material without written permission from the publisher.

89

AOS programs typically note psychiatric problems and document the effects of those problems on a patient's addiction treatment plan. To move to the DDC level, an AOS program must address a patient's psychiatric problem by at least implementing generic interventions such as cognitive-behavioral therapy for substance use, feelings or anger management groups, and individual counseling. At this level, these treatments may be more clinician-driven than program-driven. DDE programs tend to have the greatest capacity and ability to incorporate psycho-social/behavioral interventions (which are evidence-based when possible) into therapies for individuals in addiction treatment programs who have psychiatric disorders.

For an MHOS program to move to the DDC level, providers will need to implement interventions that address substance use, at least as a generic symptom undermining progress on the mental health disorder.

To move to the DDE level, any DDC program, whether addiction treatment or mental health, will need to develop specialized and targeted interventions and psychosocial treatments for patients with co-occurring disorders. In addiction treatment settings, these approaches may include specific manual-guided treatments for diagnosed disorders: seeking safety for PTSD, dialectical behavior therapy–substance abuse (DBT–S) for borderline personality disorder, integrated group therapy for bipolar disorder, or modified therapeutic community (MTC) for antisocial personality disorders. In mental health settings, specific evidence-based treatments for substance use disorders may be implemented. Examples of these include MET, CBT, relapse prevention therapy (RPT), or TSF. (Curriculum ❷ *Integrating Combined Therapies* incorporates MET, CBT, and TSF approaches, adapts each for stage-wise application, and can be used as DDE-level specialized interventions in either addiction treatment or mental health treatment settings. This curriculum can be delivered in either group or individual settings.)

Training is widely available in most of these manual-guided interventions, and in some regions, certified trainers and supervisors exist. Often DDE programs recognize the need for specifically targeted treatments for the most prevalent disorders (mood, anxiety, PTSD) and address this within the context of individual psychotherapy or a well-delivered cognitive-behavioral therapy group that targets both the substance use and the psychiatric disorder at the same time. These latter approaches are most typical of DDE programs, due to program size, staff resources, and the unnecessary burden of multiple manuals specific for each disorder.

Patient Education

Do your program's patient educational components include information about psychiatric disorders and addiction treatment, or substance use and mental health treatment?

Patient education, from diabetes to dental health, is believed to be associated with treatment engagement, compliance, and outcomes. Addiction treatment has a long history of educating patients about the physical, mental, and spiritual aspects of the disease, and has recognized the importance of patient knowledge in appreciating the scope of the task at hand. At first glance, the solution to addiction—not drinking or using—is an obvious and simple one. However, given the biological, psychological, and social aspects of an individual's attachment to alcohol or drugs, this task is anything but easy.

Most addiction treatment programs have an excellent addiction education curricula built into a patient's treatment experience. Although there is awareness that knowledge and education are helpful as adjuncts, they are not in and of themselves therapeutic. Nonetheless, in residential programs and intensive out-patient programs, patient education may constitute at least one hour per week. Group and/or individual counseling may also be used to educate patients about the nature and process of addiction. Impaired driver programs also rely heavily on patient education.

Integrating curricula on psychiatric disorders in addiction treatment would add to patients' knowledge base and aid them in their formidable challenge of recovery from co-occurring disorders. Patients should learn about the relationship between substance use and a psychiatric disorder, the role of medication, how to utilize professionals in recovery, and how to connect with peer group supports.

Mental health treatment providers have likewise utilized patient education to support the care of psychiatric disorders. This is particularly done with pharmacological and CBT approaches. Mental health providers can augment their services by educating patients about substance use disorders.

Use the Facts Sheets on common disorders found in curricula ❷, ❸, and ❺ to educate patients.

Duplicating this page is illegal. Do not copy this material without written permission from the publisher.

91

Evaluate Your Patient Education

To evaluate your program's patient education on co-occurring disorders, review your program's schedules of psychoeducational groups and educational components and ask if both mental health and substance use disorders and their interactive course are included in treatment information.

Improve Your Patient Education

It's important to educate patients about the nature of addiction and mental health disorders as a disease. Patients should understand the effects co-occurring disorders have on the family, and they should also understand the role of treatment and peer recovery support groups in long-term recovery. AOS programs typically take this approach, but focus only on the aspects related to substance use and not psychiatric disorders. To move to the DDC level, AOS programs must also offer educational components focused on psychiatric disorders. This can be accomplished

---

Evaluate an Addiction Treatment Program

*In general, an addiction treatment program's **patient education materials** will fall into one of these four categories.*

The program will

- focus educational components on substance use disorders and not on psychiatric disorders. Educational components do not educate patients on the interaction between substance use and psychiatric disorders.

- focus educational components primarily on substance use disorders, and occasionally on psychiatric disorders and mental health treatment, but only as these issues relate to substance use disorders and concerns.

- regularly focus educational components on both substance use disorders and psychiatric disorders and their interactions. These educational components are, however, meant only to provide information about psychiatric disorders and are not designed to be treatment techniques. Examples include a general orientation to co-occurring disorders, educational lectures about psychiatric disorders and mental health symptoms, and educational lectures about the connections between mental health symptoms and substance use, as well as the appropriate use of psychotropic medications.

- regularly offer a combination of general education components that address both disorders and describe interventions such as cognitive-behavioral therapy, feelings or anger management groups, and individual counseling. These comprehensive educational components target specific issues relating to the interaction between substance use and mental health. Topics might include the interaction between alcohol and marijuana use and social anxiety.

through group therapy or community meetings, or through family sessions and/or individual sessions. These offerings may be fairly generic and driven by clinician preferences but are a vast improvement to offering nothing on the subject. In a similar way, MHOS programs can move to the DDC level by offering educational components focused on how substances affect mental health problems and treatment.

To move to the DDE level, DDC programs should implement a more systematic approach to delivering information about co-occurring disorders. A program schedule should illustrate that patients receive information on both types of disorders and how the disorders interact. Patients should be made aware that long-term healing for both disorders is possible when the patient maintains long-term engagement in treatment and with recovery supports. The materials available for these didactics should be carefully prepared and used consistently according to the program protocol and not just by clinician preference.

Evaluate a Mental Health Treatment Program

*In general, a mental health treatment program's **patient education materials** will fall into one of these four categories.*

The program will

- focus educational components on mental health disorders and not on substance use disorders or the interaction with substance use disorders. Educational components do not educate patients on the interaction between psychiatric disorders and substance use.

- focus educational components primarily on mental health disorders, and occasionally on substance use disorders and addiction treatment, but only as these issues relate to psychiatric disorders and concerns.

- regularly focus educational components on both substance use disorders and psychiatric disorders and their interactions. These educational components are, however, meant only to provide information about substance use disorders and are not designed to be treatment techniques. Examples include a general orientation to co-occurring disorders, educational lectures about the disease of addiction, and educational lectures about the connections between substance use and mental health symptoms, as well as information about anti-addiction medications.

- regularly offer a combination of general education components that address both disorders and describe interventions such as cognitive-behavioral therapy, feelings or anger management groups, and individual counseling. These comprehensive educational components target specific issues relating to the interaction between mental health and substance use. Topics might include the interaction between alcohol and marijuana use and social anxiety.

Facts Sheets are available for patients and include general information about co-occurring disorders, bipolar disorder, dysthymia, generalized anxiety disorder, major depression, obsessive-compulsive disorder, panic disorder, PTSD, schizoaffective disorder, schizophrenia, and social anxiety disorder. (The sheets are available in curricula ❷, ❸, and ❺ of the Co-occurring Disorders Program.)

Each sheet describes characteristics of the disorder, explains what the disorder "is not," and lists the primary symptoms, causes, and usual treatments for the disorder. The sheets also give information regarding the effects of drugs and alcohol on the disorder and how the disorder affects treatment and recovery from addictions. The sheets also include information on treatment for co-occurring mental health and substance use disorders.

Patient Education Resources

Some excellent materials to improve patient education are available from the Substance Abuse and Mental Health Services Administration (SAMHSA), National Institute of Mental Health (NIMH), and Center for Mental Health Services (CMHS) Web sites.

 See the CD-ROM included with this guidebook for links to these sites.

Family Education

In your program, is family education and support offered? A considerable number—if not the majority—of phone calls an addiction treatment program receives are from family members concerned about a loved one in treatment or a loved one whom they would like to get into treatment. Wise addiction treatment programs attempt to harness this interest by offering family information sessions for prospective patients and family sessions, including education and therapeutic aspects, for existing patients.

Families, broadly defined here as any interested collateral party, can be the single most important resource or contaminant to recovery. As Alan Marlatt's

 Utilize the Co-occurring Disorders Program DVD, *A Guide for Living with Co-occurring Disorders*, as an excellent source of education for patients and their family.

work suggests, although negative emotion is identified as the number one relapse trigger, more often than not, the negative emotion is secondary to relationship issues (Marlatt & Gordon, 1985). Attending to these relationships in addiction treatment, and engaging the key people from the patient's social environment, is an excellent practice.

Many addiction treatment programs, particularly those in the private sector, have developed family services components. In the public sector, family services are more mixed, in part due to the demand in offering these services, but this also may be associated with the belief that patients have destroyed their support systems and are essentially isolated. This belief is not fully supported by the data from public sector programs.

Nonetheless, the existence of family service programs is a variable in all of addiction treatment and perhaps all of health care. Your program's ability to offer integrated treatment for co-occurring disorders will be enhanced with a treatment program that involves and educates interested family members.

In considering this benchmark, the assumption is that an educated and supportive family will result in better outcomes for patients with co-occurring disorders. While family members may or may not be educated about substance use and recovery issues, they are often not informed about the interaction between addiction and mental health problems. Family members should be educated about the causes of these disorders, the treatments for both disorders, and what is required to ensure long-term recovery. Families need basic information about medication use, types of treatment services needed, the dangers of a patient not taking his or her medication, and the negative effects of drinking or using drugs while taking prescription medication. Often families and patients lack basic information about these issues. When family members are educated and supportive, treatment can proceed smoothly, which only improves patient (and family) outcomes.

Program Resources

Utilize the Co-occurring Disorders Program DVD, *A Guide for Living with Co-occurring Disorders*, which offers clinicians expert guidance on the importance of creating and executing a family program to support treatment. Also use curriculum ❺ *Family Program*.

Evaluate Your Family Education Services

To learn about your program's family education services, review your educational and supportive materials for the family or significant others. Do these materials address co-occurring disorders? Determine if these components feature both types of disorders and if they explain how each disorder affects the other. (See the box at the bottom of this page and on page 97 to evaluate an addiction or mental health treatment program.)

Improve Your Family Education Services

Treatment of patients with co-occurring disorders is enhanced when family members and significant others are educated on and involved in treatment. AOS programs typically offer family education focused on substance use but not on mental health issues. To move to the DDC level, AOS programs must begin to incorporate mental health education for family members into the treatment plan. These types of educational components may still be clinician-driven more than program-driven. An MHOS program may typically offer family members education on mental health disorders but not on substance use disorders. MHOS programs

---

Evaluate an Addiction Treatment Program

*In general, a program's **family education literature** falls into one of these five categories.*

The program

- focuses education and support for family members and significant others on substance use disorders only.

- occasionally focuses education and support for family members and significant others on psychiatric disorders as needed. These components are typically informal and are based on the expertise of the clinician.

- routinely focuses education and support for family members and significant others on co-occurring disorders. Though many families may access this service, it is not considered to be a standard part of the routine program format.

- routinely focuses education and support for family members and significant others on co-occurring disorders. Education and support are then incorporated into intervention and recovery plans.

- routinely focuses education and support for family members and significant others on co-occurring disorders. This is a standard part of the treatment intervention with families and members of support systems, meaning that a majority of families of individuals with co-occurring disorders participate in these activities.

can move to the DDC level by including family education on substance use and addiction treatment as part of the patient's treatment plan.

For any program to move to the DDE level, the educational components must be systematic and part of an overall program schedule with focus on interactive risks of co-occurring disorders. Careful discussions about drugs versus medications, chronic versus acute care models, and the importance of family support should be routinely conducted.

SAMHSA's *Family Psychoeducation: Implementation Resource Kit* offers information on family education and support programming. Visit www.mentalhealth.samhsa.gov for more information.

See the CD-ROM included with this guidebook for a direct link.

Also utilize curriculum ❺ *Family Program* and the DVD entitled *A Guide for Living with Co-occurring Disorders.*

Evaluate a Mental Health Treatment Program

*In general, a program's **family education literature** falls into one of these five categories.* The program

- focuses education and support for family members and significant others on mental health disorders only.

- occasionally focuses education and support for family members and significant others on substance use disorders as needed. These components are typically informal and are based on the expertise of the clinician.

- routinely focuses education and support for family members and significant others on co-occurring disorders. Though many families may access this service, it is not considered to be a standard part of the routine program format.

- routinely focuses education and support for family members and significant others on co-occurring disorders. Education and support are then incorporated into intervention and recovery plans.

- routinely focuses education and support for family members and significant others on co-occurring disorders. This is a standard part of the treatment intervention with families and members of support systems, meaning that a majority of families of individuals with co-occurring disorders participate in these activities.

Specialized Interventions for Peer Support

Does your program use specialized interventions to facilitate the use of peer recovery support groups? The cornerstone of much of traditional addiction treatment continues to be the power of peer support, particularly through established groups such as Alcoholics Anonymous (AA), Narcotics Anonymous (NA), and Dual Recovery Anonymous (DRA).

These groups, with origins dating back at least seventy years, have provided fellowship, a program of action, and a spiritual connection that are evidenced-based and associated with long-term recovery.

The tradition of peer support philosophy and practice in addiction treatment has been under fire in recent years. This is due to demands for practices to be more science- and medicine-based. In addition, there has been a growing awareness that more than one road to recovery should be offered to patients suffering from substance use disorders. Related to this is the finding that many patients, perhaps due to the other problems from which they suffer, may not easily embrace, fit, or benefit from peer recovery support groups.

As addiction treatment has evolved, most programs have become more multi-faceted. They continue to vary on the role of peer support and Twelve Step group philosophy. Some programs believe in simple exposure: "We want to introduce our patients to this model and approach as *one* option." Others take a unifying approach: "We see the Twelve Step approach as the best available vehicle to make lifelong and real changes from addiction." Nonetheless, each of these programs can agree that patients with co-occurring disorders may have particular challenges in connecting with peers and in feeling comfortable enough to stick with Twelve Step recovery groups.

Programs can consider developing their facilitation to peer support curriculum so that some attention to co-occurring disorders is a feature. For instance, for

---

Program Resources

Curriculum ❷ *Integrating Combined Therapies* includes an adaptation of TSF that can be added to adaptations of motivational enhancement therapy (MET) and cognitive-behavioral therapy (CBT) for a combined stage-wise approach to co-occurring disorders in addiction treatment. Treatment programs can use this guide to enhance their capability to offer integrated treatment for co-occurring disorders.

---

patients suffering from depression, it may be important to know about the nature of depressive symptoms, which may pose challenges to "working the Steps." Patients with bipolar disorder may need to learn how to share appropriately at meetings and discover the limits of personal disclosure beyond problems with drugs or alcohol.

Two existing evidence-based practices on the benefits of peer group support exist for persons with substance use disorders. These are Twelve Step facilitation (TSF) and individual or group drug counseling (IDC or GDC). Although these practices are not specific to persons with co-occurring disorders, they can be adapted with this population in mind.

Other options include increasing the number of types of peer recovery support groups offered and supported by your program. Specific groups for co-occurring disorders, such as DRA or Double Trouble in Recovery (DTR), may be helpful for patients with co-occurring disorders. These kinds of groups, in addition to more careful and intentional facilitation of connection to the longer-standing peer recovery support groups, such as AA and NA, are an excellent resource to patients over the longer-term course of their recovery.

Evaluate an Addiction or Mental Health Treatment Program

*In general, an AOS or MHOS program's **peer recovery support** falls into one of these four categories.*

The program

- does not link patients with co-occurring disorders to peer recovery support groups.

- occasionally links patients with co-occurring disorders with appropriate peer recovery support groups, but this is usually based on the clinician's judgment or preference.

- regularly links individuals with co-occurring disorders with appropriate peer recovery support groups by providing schedules of these groups and some initial contacts made on behalf of the individual.

- systematically links individuals with co-occurring disorders with appropriate peer recovery support groups. This information is documented in the patient's treatment plan. In addition, the program proactively anticipates potential barriers or difficulties that the client might experience in the peer recovery support group environment. The clinician identifies a liaison to assist the patient in transitioning to the support group and provides consultation (regarding specialized mental health or addiction treatment needs) with the support group on behalf of the patient. The clinician may offer an on-site "transition group" that includes support group members who are willing to discuss co-occurring disorders.

Evaluate Your Specialized Interventions for Peer Support

Evaluate your program's approach to peer recovery supports for persons with co-occurring disorders by reviewing recovery plans to determine if your program provides a support system for patients through in-house peer recovery support groups or by linking to outside groups. Individuals with mental health symptoms and substance use disorders often face significant barriers in linking with peer recovery support groups. These patients require additional assistance, such as being referred or introduced to a peer recovery support group. A member of the clinical staff, a designated liaison, or a peer volunteer (buddy) may need to accompany the patient to the first group meeting.

Improve Your Specialized Interventions for Peer Support

Peer recovery support groups are typically very beneficial to individuals with co-occurring disorders. The members of these groups provide a solid support system

---

Dual Recovery Resources

- Dual Recovery Anonymous (www.draonline.org) and Double Trouble in Recovery (www.doubletroubleinrecovery.org) are the most common peer recovery support groups designed specifically for people with co-occurring disorders.

- Hazelden has produced a 30-minute DVD entitled *Introduction to Twelve Step Groups* and *The Twelve Step Facilitation Outpatient Program* based on TSF. Visit hazelden.org/bookstore for more information.

- There are two standardized, evidence-based methods of connecting with peer group support in the community:

  —NIDA Therapy Manuals for Individual Drug Counseling and Group Drug Counseling

  —NIAAA Therapy Component for Twelve Step Facilitation Therapy (TSF)

  Although neither of these approaches specifically addresses co-occurring psychiatric barriers, they can be adapted for this purpose.

  See the CD-ROM included with this guidebook for direct links to these resources.

- Also utilize curriculum ❷ *Integrating Combined Therapies* as a specialized intervention to facilitate connection to peer recovery supports.

---

of fellow non-users and acknowledge the vulnerabilities of lifelong addiction. These groups also provide systematic approaches and guidelines for change. Sometimes individuals with co-occurring disorders find these groups difficult to adjust to; for this reason, groups specific to co-occurring disorders, such as DTR and DRA, have been developed.

AOS and MHOS programs often do not link patients with co-occurring disorders to traditional peer recovery support groups. DDC programs may make efforts to link patients to a peer recovery support group by providing informational sessions and in-house meetings. These are often clinician-driven and are not standard procedure.

A program seeking to move to the DDE level should promote co-occurring disorder recovery groups on-site and should systematically address the possible challenges patients face when dealing with specific co-occurring disorders. These may include helping a person with depression learn about the role of medications in recovery and how to (or not) discuss medicines in groups. A clinician may need to help a patient with social phobia gradually approach a peer recovery support group, first by attending smaller groups, then by showing up earlier and staying later to minimize public speaking anxiety. A clinician may need to help a person with PTSD find a "safe" meeting that will not likely cause the patient to re-experience PTSD symptoms. These interventions may be conducted within the context of a co-occurring disorder group and may feature clinicians attending meetings with patients in order to facilitate affiliation. DDE programs document the various strategies used to help people connect with peer recovery support groups to share across all staff and retain the knowledge when staff turnover occurs.

Co-occurring disorder recovery groups should be utilized when possible. In the absence of such groups, DDE programs should use intentional and routine facilitation approaches to AA and NA groups for medication, anxiety, avoidance, sponsorship, and speaking challenges common among people with co-occurring disorders.

The book *Cognitive-Behavioral Therapy for Specific Problems and Populations* is an excellent reference for CBT groups for depression, anxiety disorders, and dual disorders.

See the CD-ROM for a link to purchase this book.

Duplicating this page is illegal. Do not copy this material without written permission from the publisher.

101

Access to Peer Recovery Role Models

Does your program offer peer recovery supports for patients with co-occurring psychiatric disorders? Addiction treatment programs have long recognized the power of recovery examples or role models in showing patients what might be possible for them. Going from the "Gift of Despair" to the "Gift of Hope" is no easy feat. It is extraordinarily powerful to be able to identify with a person of a similar gender, background, and experience. There is the "I want what she has!" factor, which is a great motivator in early recovery and perhaps throughout all of recovery.

Although not articulated, one must also assume that identification is also important for the person with a co-occurring disorder. Enhanced healing can happen when a patient can identify—through gender, ethnicity, family of origin culture, or even profession—with another person who has achieved long-term recovery.

Some programs have built upon this principle by forming alumni groups or an advisory council. Members in these groups return to the active program and have small group discussions, lectures, or informal meetings with existing patients. Certain programs formalize these sessions and call them "bridge" groups and use the time for question-and-answer sessions about the basics of peer group recovery, especially using AA groups for recovery. More enhanced treatment programs have developed alumni or peer support "mentors" who engage patients with co-occurring disorders. If your program decides to offer on-site peer recovery supports that can

Evaluate an Addiction or Mental Health Treatment Program

*In general, an AOS or MHOS program's access to **peer recovery role models** falls into one of these five categories.*

The program

- does not utilize peer supports or role models in treatment plans for individuals with co-occurring disorders.
- occasionally refers individuals to off-site peer recovery support groups, but this is based on clinician preferences and knowledge of available peer recovery support groups in the area.
- routinely refers individuals to off-site peer recovery support groups or links them with role models as part of a standard service protocol.
- routinely integrates off-site peer supports into the recovery plan for individuals with co-occurring disorders.
- routinely offers peer supports on-site. These peer supports are consistently integrated and documented in recovery plans.

be matched to individual patients, you will enhance your treatment services and the outlook for patient recovery.

Evaluate Your Access to Peer Recovery Role Models

Evaluate your program's performance on this benchmark by reviewing the available peer recovery supports that are on-site as well as consumer liaisons and alumni groups. The next step is to ask if individuals in your program are encouraged to use these peer recovery support groups and other role models as part of their treatment.

Improve Your Access to Peer Recovery Role Models

AOS and MHOS programs typically do not link individuals with co-occurring disorders to peer supports or role models. To move to the DDC level, these programs should encourage staff members to make special introductions to peer supports or meetings on behalf of the individual. Clinicians can "match" individuals with temporary sponsors, even if this is done informally.

To move to the DDE level, DDC programs must routinely and systematically match individuals with peer mentors or supports on-site. This match can be based on mental health disorders in the patient's background and the need to learn how to live with both mental health and substance use disorders. Volunteer boards, program alumni, Twelve Step Hospital and Institution Committees (HIC), or bridging the gap groups are quality resources for matching.

The establishment of weekly "bridge" groups, which are co-led by recovering volunteers and a staff member and have a segment dedicated to co-occurring psychiatric issues, is the way some successful treatment centers have responded to this crucial issue.

•   •   •

Duplicating this page is illegal. Do not copy this material without written permission from the publisher.

103

Clinical Practice: Evaluating Continuity of Care

Chapter 8 covers continuity of care as the final chapter in evaluating how the clinical practices of your program affect your capacity to offer integrated treatment for people with co-occurring disorders.

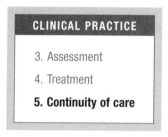

CLINICAL PRACTICE

3. Assessment

4. Treatment

5. Continuity of care

Continuity of care encompasses five benchmarks that directly address the chronic care and recovery model approach, both of which are understood as evidence-based and consistent with a realistic and enlightened approach to treatment for persons with co-occurring disorders.

In the sections that follow, the five continuity of care benchmarks are defined in detail, and examples of programs that are operating at DDC and DDE levels are given. Suggestions for how a program may consider enhancing its performance on each benchmark are also noted.

Understanding Your Program's Continuity of Care

In a classic article entitled "Drug Dependence, a Chronic Medical Illness" in the *Journal of the American Medical Association,* McLellan and colleagues compared the course of substance use disorders to that of diabetes, hypertension, and asthma (McLellan et al., 2000). The review revealed that addiction is similar to other chronic diseases with regard to etiology, relapse rate, the role of personal responsibility in symptom management, and recidivism. This article helped to realistically contextualize addiction as a chronic relapsing condition for which brief acute care treatments have important but not curative effects. Therefore, treatment for addiction is best understood using a long-term perspective that offers more intense treatment methods during acutely symptomatic episodes, and less intense (but still available) treatment during periods of relative stability. Medications, periodic checkups, family support, and peer recovery supports to "normalize" life adjustment and coping are all protective factors that have been shown to improve long-term recovery outcomes.

Duplicating this page is illegal. Do not copy this material without written permission from the publisher.

105

Of course, treating addiction the same as other chronic diseases is a concept that has been understood for decades by many in personal recovery, if not by the insurance and health care industries. Nonetheless, research is now discovering the veracity of this approach, as well as comprehensive health programs within medication-assisted recovery clinics.

Psychiatric disorders are also best understood as chronic conditions that will at least require periodic monitoring if not lifelong care. Once affected, a person remains at risk even after extended periods of relative stability. Relapse is common though not inevitable. Persons in recovery from psychiatric problems have also grown increasingly appreciative of peer recovery supports and a shift from symptom management to having a life worth living.

CONTINUITY OF CARE BENCHMARKS

Continuity of care refers to five specific benchmarks that should be evaluated in this order:

1. Discharge planning
2. Treatment continuity
3. Dual recovery focus
4. Peer recovery support in the community
5. Medication management

For both substance use and mental health disorders, many recovery models are now based on improving the patient's quality of life—not just seeking to remove the disease. Addiction treatment programs have historically focused on recovery and relapse issues with respect to substance use. Mental health providers have focused on mental health symptoms, and a relapse meant a return to a negative state of mental health—which could also lead to an increased desire to use alcohol or other drugs as a coping mechanism.

The chronic disease model of care and the recovery model for co-occurring disorders have required treatment programs to shift from short-term acute care models to longer-term perspectives. The relationship between mental health and substance use problems is not understood as one directional, but rather is bi-directional, such that both will simultaneously need to be addressed at discharge and over time.

Discharge Planning

Does your program address co-occurring disorders in the discharge planning process?

Acute care models, such as detoxification programs, and even some short-term residential addiction treatment programs (e.g., the twenty-eight-day program) have developed treatment and discharge plans as if all the important changes in a person's life take place during this time period. Unfortunately, there is no evidence that even the most dramatic changes in residential, detoxification, or hospital settings are associated with adjustment in community settings. For this reason, the focus must be on the discharge plan and on solidifying supports and connections at the community and home level. Outpatient treatment programs, often time-limited, must also consider the plan for treatment or recovery beyond the regular meeting phase. Of course, a good connection with community peer recovery support groups may naturalistically assist with this process; however, what are the mechanisms for the patient to continue to be monitored by a professional? By what process will the patient be involved in recovery checkups, both for mental health and substance-related problems?

Recovery rates for addicted professionals, although not studied within randomized controlled trials, show higher two- and five-year abstinence rates (80 percent or more) than abstinence rates in community treatment (approximately 20 percent). Many believe it is the resources of the professional population that account for these outcome differences. Others believe that it is the quality and amount of treatment that addicted professionals have access to and the long-term, regular monitoring that result in higher rates of abstinence. Physicians in recovery have reported that long-term, regular monitoring is the most important factor in a successful recovery.

At discharge, adjustment to the "real world" officially begins, so it is imperative to create a plan to continue to address the patient's ongoing mental health and substance use problems. These plans should be transparent between provider and patient. They should also be established with regard to the patient's stage of motivation to change and treatment readiness. The process that allows the patient to proceed to this next level of care must be clear-cut and simple. A discharge plan, from an acute episode in treatment, is best if it has a coherent and balanced plan to address both the mental health and substance use disorder.

A detoxification program on the East Coast transfers men from their clinically managed setting to an affiliated addiction treatment program and a coordinated local mental health clinic. Prior to discharge, staff members arrange for the initial patient appointment and a primary caregiver accompanies the patient to the first appointment. When the patient is discharged from detoxification services, he has already visited his outpatient program (for addiction and mental health) and met his counselor. This has improved linkage to both programs and addresses both substance use and mental health problems with equivalence.

Duplicating this page is illegal. Do not copy this material without written permission from the publisher.

107

Evaluate Your Discharge Planning

To evaluate your program's performance on this benchmark, review your documented discharge plans and medical records to determine if the focus is placed equally on follow-up services for both mental health and substance use disorders. As with all other benchmark items, it is important to identify whether discharge plans are defined by protocol or are variable by the preference of individual clinicians. The best programs approach and utilize discharge plans in a systematic, routine manner, and these plans are guided by formats in the medical record or emergency medical record. (See the box at the bottom of this page and on page 109 to evaluate an addiction or mental health treatment program's discharge planning.)

Improve Your Discharge Planning

AOS programs typically do not include co-occurring psychiatric disorders in treatment plans; for this reason, treatment of psychiatric disorders is not included in discharge plans. Similarly, MHOS programs do not include co-occurring substance use disorders in treatment plans; for this reason, addiction treatment is not included in discharge plans.

To move to the DDC level, AOS and MHOS programs must acknowledge the influence of co-occurring disorders on one another. Though one disorder might

---

Evaluate an Addiction Treatment Program

*In general, an addiction treatment program's **discharge plans** fall into one of these five categories.*

The program

- routinely focuses only on substance use disorders and not on mental health concerns.

- occasionally addresses both the substance use disorder and the psychiatric disorder, depending on an individual clinician's judgment or preference.

- routinely addresses both the substance use disorder and the psychiatric disorder, but significant emphasis is placed on the substance use disorder. Follow-up mental health services are managed through outside agencies, or are generically addressed as part of the relapse (substance) prevention plan.

- occasionally plans for integrated follow-up that equally addresses substance use and psychiatric disorders.

- routinely addresses both the substance use disorder and the psychiatric disorder. Both disorders are included in follow-up plans in-house or with outside agencies as defined in a formal agreement.

---

be considered primary, treatments for the other disorder (pharmacological and psychosocial) should be included in discharge plans. Collaborative relationships with providers play an important role in recovery and should be addressed in the discharge plan.

To move to the DDE level, DDC programs must create systematic, program-driven discharge plans that focus equally on substance use and psychiatric disorders. Treatment providers and interventions, medications and doses, recovery supports, and relapse risks for both disorders should be well described and documented.

Treatment Continuity

Does your program provide continuity of treatment? Some people feel that next to choosing a partner for marriage, the most important choice we make in life is in choosing a therapist. Although this may strike some as hyperbole, few would argue that the attachment patients make with a treatment provider is a critically important and potentially enduring one. Many patients will disclose things to a therapist that they have never spoken about before. This can include a history of childhood sexual abuse and/or an adulthood of leading a double life as a functional citizen and as a raging drug addict. They tell this story for the first time, expecting shame and reprobation and instead receive applause, if not understanding. Having

---

Evaluate a Mental Health Treatment Program

*In general, a mental health treatment program's **discharge plans** fall into one of these five categories.*

The program

- routinely focuses only on mental health disorders and not on substance use concerns.

- occasionally addresses both the psychiatric disorder and the substance use disorder, but varies depending on an individual clinician's judgment or preference.

- routinely addresses both the psychiatric disorder and the substance use disorder, but significant emphasis is placed on the psychiatric disorder. Follow-up addiction treatment services are managed through outside agencies, or are generically addressed as part of the relapse (mental health) prevention plan.

- occasionally plans for integrated follow-up that equally addresses psychiatric disorders and substance use disorders.

- routinely addresses both the psychiatric disorder and the substance use disorder. Both disorders are included in follow-up plans in-house or with outside agencies as defined in a formal agreement.

just developed trust in a treatment provider, they learn that moving on is a necessary part of the treatment process.

Nonetheless, particularly in outpatient settings, continuity of care is possible and time-unlimited treatment is an option. There may be some realistic limitations to the amount of contact a patient has with his or her former therapist based on managed care, staff caseload, or other considerations, but recovery checkups may be considered routine care.

In hospital or residential settings, continuity of care with the patient's existing treatment provider may be less realistic. Nonetheless, clearly defined linkage to the next level of care is imperative. Some residential programs have built in return visits for patients. These can include peer support group meetings, alumni weekends, or events to reinforce continuity. Other residential programs have developed or are connected to outpatient components and have some clinical staff, such as a physician or psychologist, who work in both the outpatient and inpatient (hospital or residential) levels of care. This common staff denominator provides a nice sense of continuity for patients who are making a transition from a structured to an unstructured environment.

Another aspect of this benchmark is the policy for patients who become psychiatrically symptomatic during the course of addiction treatment. Are these patients treated within the addiction treatment program until stabilized? Are they referred for psychiatric care, and once stabilized are they accepted back into the addiction treatment program? Or once they become psychiatrically symptomatic are they forever "blacklisted" from addiction treatment services for fear that these symptoms will return?

Also consider the policy for substance use relapse in mental health treatment programs. How does the mental health treatment program respond to substance use? Are these patients treated within the mental health treatment program until stabilized? Are they referred for addiction treatment and once stabilized are they accepted back into the mental health program? Or are they forever "blacklisted" from the mental health treatment program once they exhibit a substance use disorder?

These questions suggest that continuity of care is not only important to consider with respect to recovery from addiction but is equally important for psychiatric recovery.

Evaluate Your Treatment Continuity

You can learn about your program's approach to continuity of care by reviewing your procedures for providing consistent follow-up care for both disorders. Ask if your program's overall goal is co-occurring disorder illness management.

Evaluate an Addiction Treatment Program

*In general, an addiction treatment program's **continuity of care**
falls into one of these four categories.*

The program

■ offers follow-up care for substance use disorders only, and not for psychiatric disorders. Follow-up for psychiatric disorders may be offered through outside agencies but with no formal consultation or collaboration.

■ offers follow-up care for substance use disorders only, and possibly for psychiatric disorders if individual clinicians are willing and capable of providing it.

■ offers continued monitoring/support for psychiatric disorders and substance use disorders. If this service is not possible, the program depends on defined relationships with outside agencies for support. This in turn ensures a rapid return for program services when needed.

■ monitors and treats both psychiatric disorders and substance use disorders over an extended or indefinite period. Recovery checkups may be an annual option in this type of program.

Evaluate a Mental Health Treatment Program

*In general, a mental health treatment program's **continuity of care**
falls into one of these four categories.*

The program

■ offers follow-up care for mental health disorders only, and not for substance use disorders. Follow-up for substance use disorders may be offered through outside agencies but with no formal consultation or collaboration.

■ offers follow-up care for mental health disorders only, and possibly for substance use disorders if individual clinicians are willing and capable of providing it.

■ offers continued monitoring/support for substance use disorders and psychiatric disorders. If this service is not possible, the program depends on defined relationships with outside agencies for support. This in turn ensures a rapid return for program services when needed.

■ monitors and treats both substance use and psychiatric disorders over an extended or indefinite period. Recovery checkups may be an annual option in this type of program.

Improve Your Treatment Continuity

AOS programs often discharge a patient with a co-occurring disorder who develops acute psychiatric symptoms. Similarly MHOS programs may discharge a patient with a co-occurring disorder who returns to alcohol or other drug use.

To move to the DDC level, AOS and MHOS programs must develop procedures for dealing with changing levels of psychiatric symptoms as well as relapses where the patient returns to alcohol or drug use. Typically, DDC programs evaluate the changing symptoms of both disorders. If the patient is sufficiently stable, the patient will be allowed to remain in the current program. If a referral is required—preferably within the same agency or to a mental health agency or addiction treatment program with whom there is a memorandum of understanding (or a charter agreement)—the program will accept the patient back once he or she is stabilized.

To move to the DDE level, DDC programs must provide in-house services to deal effectively with changing levels of psychiatric and substance use symptoms or relapses indefinitely.

Dual Recovery Focus

Does your program focus on ongoing recovery issues for both mental health and substance use disorders? Since recovery from both addiction and mental health problems is a lifelong process (at least for the foreseeable future), it is imperative that patients understand the breadth and scope of recovery.

Programs offering integrated or enhanced services for persons with co-occurring disorders focus on the dual recovery aspect with equanimity. These programs inspire patients with hope for the future. "You are not alone" is a key take-home message for patients.

People in recovery from substance use often are able to find support from peers who openly share their common experience in struggling with and recovering from the disease of addiction. In contrast, it can be harder for people with psychiatric disorders to find peer support, although the outlets for these recovery supports are increasing. Peer support is imperative in helping patients deal with the stigma of both addiction and psychiatric disorders. The type and intensity of stigma a patient encounters varies from community to community, from culture to culture, and from person to person. Programs that address this issue within the treatment plan will help a patient feel like less of an outcast and more "normal."

Evaluate Your Dual Recovery Focus

In considering your program's approach to this benchmark, you will need to review your program practices, which can often be found in discharge plans and via conversations with staff and patients. Review these materials and ask if the concept of recovery (versus remission) is used in the treatment and planning for both substance use and psychiatric disorders. In talking with current and past patients in the program, ask: "How was your recovery discussed, planned, and envisioned? Did we address both your mental health and substance use issues for the long term?"

Improve Your Dual Recovery Focus

AOS programs typically focus on recovery from addiction with little or no attention paid to psychiatric disorders. These AOS programs take traditional approaches such as aftercare, Twelve Step group affiliation, sponsorship, and remaining abstinent one day at a time. These methods are effective; however, an individual with co-occurring disorders needs to receive attention for his or her mental health concerns as well. Therefore, to move to the DDC level, AOS programs' treatment plans must address how psychiatric problems complicate or are risk factors to a patient's recovery from addiction. The treatment plan should address the importance

---

Evaluate an Addiction Treatment Program

*In general, the **dual recovery focus** of an addiction treatment program falls into one of these four categories.*

The program focuses on

- substance use disorders only. Mental health recovery is not incorporated.

- substance use disorders only, unless there are individual clinicians who use recovery focus when planning services for mental health disorders as well.

- substance use disorders with some inclusion of a dual recovery focus for co-occurring psychiatric disorders as these disorders impact recovery from the substance use disorder. For example, if it is believed that untreated mental health issues could trigger a relapse of the substance use disorder, then the mental health issues will be included in treatment. In addition, mental health issues may be considered to be part of generic wellness and positive lifestyle change.

- recovery from both substance use and psychiatric disorders equally, and the program articulates specific goals to achieve and maintain recovery from both mental health and substance use disorders.

---

of medication compliance, include attendance at cognitive-behavioral therapy sessions, or perhaps involve collaboration with a community mental health center's case management staff members.

Similarly, MHOS programs typically focus on recovery from psychiatric symptoms with no or little attention paid to substance use disorders. These MHOS programs take traditional approaches such as medications, professional support, and cognitive-behavioral therapy.

These methods are effective; however, an individual with a co-occurring disorder needs to receive attention for his or her substance use as well. To move to the DDC level, MHOS programs' treatment plans must address how substance use problems complicate or are risk factors to a patient's recovery from a psychiatric disorder. The treatment plan should address the importance of medication compliance, include cognitive-behavioral therapy for both disorders, and involve collaboration with a local addiction treatment center.

To move to the DDE level, any program must equally recognize both substance use and mental health disorders. The end goal for a DDE program is to create an environment where patients see the possibility of a new life filled with hope, promise, and opportunity for recovery from both mental health and substance use disorders. To get there, the program (and the patient) must recognize that recovery

---

Evaluate a Mental Health Treatment Program

*In general, the **dual recovery focus** of a mental health treatment program falls into one of these four categories.*

The program focuses on

- psychiatric disorders only. Addiction recovery is not incorporated.
- psychiatric disorders only, unless there are individual clinicians who use recovery focus when planning services for substance use disorders as well.
- psychiatric disorders with some inclusion of a dual recovery focus for co-occurring substance use disorders as these disorders impact recovery from the psychiatric disorder. For example, if it is believed that untreated substance use issues could trigger an increase in psychiatric symptoms, then the substance use disorder will be included in the treatment plan. In addition, substance use issues may be considered to be part of generic wellness and positive lifestyle change.
- recovery from both psychiatric and substance use disorders equally, and the program articulates specific goals to achieve and maintain recovery from both mental health and substance use disorders.

from both addiction and mental health disorders requires positive lifestyle changes and personal transformation.

Dual Recovery Focus Resource

A program's dual recovery focus must equally recognize both substance use and mental health disorders. This can be accomplished by applying Twelve Step methodology and mental health recovery literature (from the National Alliance on Mental Illness [NAMI]). Also consider using the *Illness Management and Recovery: Implementation Resource Kit* from SAMHSA.

See the link on the CD-ROM included with this guidebook.

Also, see curriculum ❷ *Integrating Combined Therapies.*

Peer Recovery Support in the Community

Does your program facilitate the connection to peer recovery support groups beyond the patient's treatment episode, out into their home community? Peer recovery supports, such as Twelve Step groups, are an excellent recovery mechanism because they are available nationwide and pose very little, if any, cost to the patient. Addiction treatment programs often have on-site peer recovery support group meetings (such as through community group commitments). They also may transport patients to and from community meetings during treatment or assign meeting attendance as homework between sessions. More enhanced addiction treatment programs take these same steps, but these programs are more systematic and intentional for persons with co-occurring disorders. For example, a program that treats female patients with PTSD will often have some developed strategies to introduce the patient to a female peer in recovery with similar comorbidity. This patient will be encouraged to attend small women-only meetings where PTSD symptoms may be explicitly discussed along with triggers and relationship issues. A patient's adjustment back into the real world after treatment is often improved when a clinician helps the patient make these peer support connections prior to discharge.

Evaluate Your Peer Recovery Support in the Community
Review the services offered by your program and determine if the program facilitates and manages connections between the patient and community peer recovery support groups. In addition, determine if the program provides the needed

assistance to support the transition to peer recovery support groups beyond active treatment. Note that programs having difficulty with the facilitation of peer recovery support groups while the individual is in treatment will also likely have difficulty meeting this benchmark when the individual is discharged.

Improve Your Peer Recovery Support in the Community

It is widely believed that continued participation in peer recovery support groups, after discharge, can lead to positive lifestyle changes and long-term success in recovery. However, AOS and MHOS programs may not have made this a primary focus of interventions or discharge plans. To move to the DDC level, AOS and MHOS programs must assist in matching individuals with community peer recovery support groups as part of the discharge plan, while making strides to encourage the development of relationships with program alumni and other non-users. To move to the DDE level, DDC programs must do this for all individuals systematically, without relying on individual clinicians to take the initiative. Current patients should always be matched with peer supports and should be accompanied to meetings to ensure a smooth transition into the group.

Evaluate an Addiction or Mental Health Treatment Program

*In general, a program's ability to connect a patient with **community-based peer support** falls into one of these five categories.*

The program

- may provide information about peer recovery support groups such as meeting lists or may suggest that the patient work the Steps or find a temporary sponsor. The program does not, however, link individuals to groups in the community.

- usually does not link individuals to community peer recovery support groups unless a clinician chooses to do so.

- frequently, but not systematically, links individuals to community peer recovery support groups at discharge. For example, women with PTSD are linked to women's peer recovery meetings or women's Twelve Step recovery meetings, such as AA or NA meetings. The program conducts a thorough discussion of medications versus drugs, including how to talk with others about co-occurring disorders and the role of prescription medication treatment.

- irregularly matches patients to peer recovery support groups in the community at discharge. This occurs at least 50 percent of the time.

- routinely links patients to peer recovery support groups in the community at discharge and recognizes that a patient may experience difficulties adjusting and may require assistance. Clinicians may introduce individuals to recovering individuals from the community, or they may accompany patients to meetings in the community or in-house.

- There are two standardized, evidence-based methods of connecting with peer group support in the community:

  —NIDA Therapy Manuals for Individual Drug Counseling and Group Drug Counseling

  —NIAAA Therapy Component for Twelve Step Facilitation Therapy (TSF)

  Although neither of these approaches specifically addresses co-occurring psychiatric barriers, they can be adapted for this purpose.

- Dual Recovery Anonymous groups and Double Trouble in Recovery groups are the most common peer recovery support groups designed specifically for people with co-occurring disorders.

  Please see the CD-ROM that accompanies this guidebook for a link to these resources.

- Also refer to "Phase III" in curriculum ❷ *Integrating Combined Therapies* for information about TSF for co-occurring disorders.

Medication Management

Does your program have a sufficient supply of and an adherence plan for prescription medications beyond the treatment episode? Since most psychiatric disorders in addiction treatment will not be cured, those patients who are prescribed and taking medications for psychiatric disorders while in addiction treatment will need to have a clear plan and mechanism to continue these medications. In some communities and regions, obtaining medication post-discharge is not difficult, particularly if the patient's financial or insurance resources are not barriers. But in other instances, providers are more scarce, and resources even scarcer. In addiction treatment centers, many patients with co-occurring disorders cannot access community mental health providers since they do not have severe and persistent mental illnesses.

Patients with severe and persistent mental illnesses typically qualify for federal or state insurance and can receive services at community mental health centers. Since many community mental health centers have lost funding, they restrict access to only persons with this public entitlement. This leaves the non-severely mentally ill person to navigate the system of primary health clinics, federally qualified health centers, free nonprofit clinics, Planned Parenthood, or, most often, hospital emergency services. Addiction treatment providers must help patients retain access to medication. If patients cannot continue their medication, they are at increased risk for psychiatric symptoms and a relapse to substance use. Patients in mental health settings may need ongoing addiction medication management for substitution (methadone, buprenorphine, and so on). It is imperative that mental health providers assist patients in continuing with these medications if clinically indicated.

Evaluate Your Medication Management

To evaluate your performance on this benchmark item, review standard discharge procedures and prescribing guidelines and determine if your program has the capacity to assist individuals with co-occurring disorders with psychotropic medication planning and prescription and medication access and monitoring. Also determine if your program is able to provide sufficient supplies of medications at discharge. Note that programs that have difficulty providing pharmacotherapy for co-occurring psychiatric disorders while the individual is in treatment will likely have difficulty providing this service at discharge.

Improve Your Medication Management

AOS programs typically do not have the capabilities to supply or manage psychiatric medications. However, these programs often link, collaborate, or consult with outside mental health agencies. To move to the DDC level, AOS programs must be able to administer and supply psychiatric medications, at least for the short-term, until a referral to an outside mental health provider has been made, has been documented, and has been successful.

Evaluate an Addiction or Mental Health Treatment Program

*In general, a program's **medication management practices** fall into one of these three categories.*

When a patient with a co-occurring disorder is discharged, the program

- may make an appointment with an outside prescriber on the individual's behalf but does not offer any medication planning or supplies.
- may offer a thirty-day supply of medications until the individual can be referred to an outside prescriber.
- provides continued medication management and prescribes medications for an indefinite period, or at least until the individual has successfully transitioned to the new care provider. In the event that the individual seeks services from an outside prescriber, the program directly collaborates with the new provider to ensure a seamless transition.

Similarly, MHOS programs typically do not have the capabilities to supply or manage addiction medications, such as naltrexone, buprenorphine, acamprosate, or disulfiram. However, these programs often link, collaborate, or consult with outside addiction treatment agencies. To move to the DDC level, MHOS programs must be aware of the current FDA-approved addiction treatment medications and be able to sustain and monitor a patient's existing medication supply, at least for the short-term, until a referral to an outside addiction treatment provider has been made, has been documented, and has been successful.

To move to the DDE level, DDC programs must be able to indefinitely prescribe and manage medications for both substance use and psychiatric disorders.

• • •

Workforce:
Evaluating Your Staff

Chapters 9 and 10 will help you evaluate your current program workforce with regard to its capacity to offer integrated treatment for people with co-occurring disorders.

This chapter focuses on staffing. Chapter 10 will complete your workforce evaluation by focusing on training.

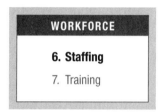

In the sections that follow, the five program staff benchmarks are defined in detail, and examples of programs that are operating at DDC and DDE levels are given. Considerations about how a program may consider enhancing its performance on each benchmark are also noted. As you evaluate your program's staff, you will investigate these five specific benchmarks, two of which are human resource based. The other three benchmarks involve the manner in which staff can be used to support effective services for patients with co-occurring disorders.

Understanding Your Program Staff

In a large survey of addiction treatment providers, respondents reported that inadequate staff preparation and expertise was one of the major barriers in providing services for patients with co-occurring disorders. This is a common perception and one that is at least partially based on reality. Some of the clinical practices in the assessment, treatment, and continuity of care dimensions definitely involve personnel who can prescribe medication.

Aspects of assessment, such as diagnosing, may also be outside the scope of practice of many counselors or clinical staff working within addiction treatment programs. The organization's leadership may be uncomfortable with nonlicensed staff providing a list of problems or "rule outs" without close supervision by a licensed clinician. Lastly, some experts may contend that cognitive-behavioral therapy is a complex psychological therapy, which can only be delivered by an appropriately trained and licensed clinician, such as a clinical psychologist or licensed clinical social worker.

PROGRAM STAFF BENCHMARKS

Program staff refers to five specific benchmarks:

1. Prescribing of medications

2. Staff expertise

3. Clinical supervision

4. Formal case review or staffings

5. On-site peer recovery support

Resolution of these concerns or restrictions can only be made within a given organization, and possibly only after that organization consults with neighboring agencies or its governing bodies to explicitly understand the exact limits to practice based on staff licensure and/or certification. Treatment programs differ on their interpretation of these guidelines, from conservative to liberal, while still operating within local laws. Some treatment providers challenge and adjust these guidelines when faced with antiquated restrictions or those that do not seem to represent the best interests of patients.

Prescribing of Medications

What type of relationship does your program have with licensed prescribing professionals? This benchmark item pertains to the role of the prescriber of medications for psychiatric disorders. Access to FDA-medications for the most common psychiatric disorders is one important (but not the only) strategy to effectively treat co-occurring disorders. Since the medications, when indicated, are likely associated with better outcomes, access to a person who can prescribe these medications is an important benchmark in the staffing dimension.

Programs vary from having no relationship with a prescriber of medications to having a clinical leader who is present for meetings, provides clinical supervision, and manages the medication needs of patients. Most often, programs will have relationships in between. Many have a consulting psychiatrist off-site, while other programs have a contractual relationship with a psychiatrist (or other prescriber) who is on-site on a limited basis.

The more "present" and involved the prescriber is, the more this person can be familiar with patient functioning and adjust medications accordingly. Most prescriptions will require some trial and error before finding the right medicine for any given patient. This challenge may be especially formidable when patients are entering periods of abstinence from alcohol and other drugs for the first time, which makes psychiatric symptoms harder to evaluate since the patients may have trouble identifying or remembering what "normal" feels like. For this reason, a prescriber with a good working knowledge, if not advanced certification, in addiction (e.g., from the American Academy of Addiction Psychiatry or American Society of

Addiction Medicine) is potentially more adept than a general psychiatric practitioner who has little training in addiction. In programs where such an expert is present, he or she serves as a clinical leader and supervisor in team meetings, rounds, or case reviews. This expanded role to support other clinical staff results in much more enhanced assessment and treatment services.

Evaluate Your Prescribing of Medications

To examine the relationship your program has with a prescriber, review the clinical treatment team of the program and determine if there is a formal relationship with a psychiatrist, physician, or nurse practitioner (or other licensed prescriber) who manages medications. This may include assesssing medication adherence or evaluating the use of potentially addictive medications such as benzodiazepines. It may also include offering medications such as disulfiram, naltrexone, or acamprosate that may be used to treat substance use disorders.

Improve Your Prescribing of Medications

For AOS and MHOS programs to move to the DDC level, they must develop formal relationships with a prescriber who can then prescribe medications and provide

---

Evaluate an Addiction or Mental Health Treatment Program

*In general, the access to a professional who can **prescribe and manage medications** falls into one of these five categories.*

The program

- cannot prescribe medications or related services for both mental health and substance use disorders and does not have a formal relationship with a prescriber.

- has an on-site medical consultant who can diagnose but does not prescribe medications for both mental health and substance use disorders. The program has made arrangements with an outside physician to prescribe medications for both disorders.

- has an on-site consultant or contractor who prescribes medications for both mental health and substance use disorders and provides related services; however, this person is not a staff member and is only available for direct patient care.

- has a prescriber on-site and on staff who prescribes medications for both mental health and substance use disorders; however, this person is not considered to be part of the clinical treatment team.

- has a prescriber on-site and on staff who prescribes medication for both mental health and substance use disorders. This person plays an active role in clinical activities and is on the clinical team, sometimes participating in decision making or serving in a supervisory role.

---

related services for substance use and psychiatric disorders. This can be accomplished by entering into a contract with a consultant. This solution may, however, not be enough to meet the needs of all patients. To move to the DDE level, a program's prescriber typically should be on-site, on staff, and heavily involved in patient care and treatment planning. The prescriber in this setting may even hold a leadership or supervisory position.

To move its program to the DDE level, the staff of one addiction treatment center in Vermont asked their consulting nurse practitioner to attend their weekly clinical team meetings. These meetings occurred every Wednesday morning. The nurse practitioner agreed to attend the meetings, which cut down on the amount of time staff needed to contact her by e-mail or phone to discuss shared patient issues. It also created an opportunity for the nurse practictioner to educate, supervise, and lead staff members, who appreciated and benefitted from this new relationship with her.

Staff Expertise

Does your program's on-site staff include individuals with mental health and substance use licensure or demonstrated mental health and substance use expertise? An increasing proportion of addiction treatment programs have masters'-level clinicians either in administrative or supervisory capacities. The availability of trained staff, many with mental health or addiction treatment license and/or certification, expands a program's potential to conduct assessments, render diagnostic impressions, and provide psychotherapeutic treatments for both disorders. Some clinicians may have more extensive expertise in addiction, while others may have more of a mental health treatment background and may be considered the "mental health person" on the addiction treatment team.

It's important that a qualified person perform patient evaluations, see individual cases as needed, and/or perhaps run a specialty treatment group. Specialty treatments include Marsha Linehan's dialectical behavior therapy (DBT), a cognitive-behavioral treatment for complex, multisystemic disorders, such as chronic suicidal behaviors and borderline personality disorder. Another specialty treatment, started by Lisa Najavits, is seeking safety: a present-focused therapy to help people attain safety from trauma/PTSD and substance use disorders. See the CD-ROM for links to Web sites about these treatments.

If your program includes a clinician licensed in addiction treatment, he or she may provide supervision or adjunctive supervision to other addiction counselor personnel. Some addiction clinicians may lack formal mental health training or licensure but have gathered considerable psychiatric treatment experience over the course of professional life. Although the determination of "expertise" is not specified, a clinician may clearly have the capacity to work with psychiatric problems, provided that he or she is supervised by a qualified staff member.

Evaluate Your Staff Expertise

In considering your staff profile, you can review the staff composition and determine the number of licensed, certified, and/or competent mental health staff members and their ability to treat co-occurring disorders.

Improve Your Staff Expertise

To move to the DDC level, AOS and MHOS programs must increase their in-house services to accommodate the treatment needs of individuals with psychiatric and substance use disorders. This can be accomplished if clinicians receive additional training and certification to be able to deliver psychosocial treatments and assessments. Training for the most basic, generic treatments should be available in your area. These may include cognitive-behavioral therapy (CBT), motivational interviewing (MI) or motivational enhancement therapy (MET), and family therapy, as well as assessments. In training staff, the program should be careful not to reduce its capability to effectively treat substance use disorders by enhancing its capacity to treat mental health disorders. When hiring clinicians, programs should seek candidates with both addiction treatment and mental health education and experience.

Evaluate an Addiction or Mental Health Treatment Program

*In general, a program's **staff composition** falls into one of these four categories.*

The program

- does not have any staff members who are capable of providing direct services to individuals with both substance use and psychiatric disorders
- has a few staff members who are capable of providing direct services to individuals with psychiatric and substance use disorders
- has many staff members who are capable of providing direct services to individuals with psychiatric and substance use disorders
- has most staff members who are capable of providing direct services to individuals with psychiatric and substance use disorders

---

To move to the DDE level, DDC programs should hire personnel who are trained and capable of assessing and providing mental health and addiction treatment. This may involve, as is in process in several states, an added qualification in co-occurring disorders. For example, Connecticut and Pennsylvania offer a co-occurring disorder specialty credential through their state certification boards. At least 50 percent of the staff should have mental health expertise. Often programs, whether residential or inpatient, at the DDE level have adequate staff/client ratios and a combination of mental health and addiction treatment staff on their second and third shifts as well.

Clinical Supervision

Does your program provide access to clinical supervision in evidence-based treatment practices for both addiction and mental health treatment? The good news is that there is considerable overlap between the evidence-based psychosocial treatments for substance use disorders (e.g., relapse prevention) and those for the most common psychiatric disorders (e.g., cognitive-behavioral therapy). Some experts believe that community addiction treatment clinicians have difficulty implementing evidence-based practices for mental health treatment due to the demands for model fidelity. Similarly, some experts feel that mental health treatment clinicians have difficulty implementing evidence-based practices for addiction treatment. Nonetheless, both mental health and addiction treatment clinicians are being increasingly trained in evidence-based approaches, such as MET, CBT, and TSF that benefit patients with co-occurring disorders. See curriculum ❷ *Integrating Combined Therapies,* which discusses MET, CBT, and TSF.

Many funding agents are now requiring some testimony that evidence-based practices are being used in patient care. Since training has not been found effective in changing or sustaining practice change, the field is presently underscoring the importance of ongoing supervision and monitoring to support and sustain any new treatment practice being implemented.

Programs with more enhanced services for persons with co-occurring disorders have established supervision protocols for staff who deliver treatments for mental health or substance use problems. Some supervision may also be focused only at the assessment and diagnostics phase of practice, whereas on the other end of the continuum, clinicians may be under supervision using component-guided treatments (e.g., CBT to treat PTSD). These supervisory relationships can also range from regular to ad hoc meetings and from discussing clinical material in depth to troubleshooting all cases. They can vary from discussing personal growth to following specific, manualized guidelines. The clinical supervisor may also be an on-site staff member or an off-site or visiting consultant.

Evaluate Your Clinical Supervision

To discover the type and level of mental health or addiction treatment supervision that exists in your program, conduct interviews with clinical supervisors. Also review staff composition and supervision structures to determine if your program offers formal supervision for mental health and addiction treatment providers who are currently unlicensed or have insufficient experience in the treatment setting. (See the box at the bottom of the page and on page 128 to evaluate an addiction or mental health treatment program's clinical supervision.)

Improve Your Clinical Supervision

For AOS programs to move to the DDC level, the programs must offer staff supervision for mental health services by a licensed professional. Similarly, MHOS programs must offer staff supervision for addiction treatment services by a licensed professional. This can be achieved on an individual or group basis and may be focused on diagnosis, referrals to prescribers, empathy, or countertransference.

To move to the DDE level, DDC programs must offer regular supervision that focuses on in-depth learning of clinical practices. These practices may include manual-guided therapies in which the agency has just received training (e.g., CBT,

---

Evaluate an Addiction Treatment Program

*In general, an addiction treatment program's **mental health treatment supervision** falls into one of these five categories.*

The program

- lacks the capacity to provide supervision for mental health treatment services.
- provides informal, irregular, and undocumented mental health supervision, usually through an off-site consultant or only in emergent situations on-site.
- offers mental health supervision on-site to staff on a semistructured basis; however, the focus is usually a crisis-management or case-disposition issue.
- offers regular, on-site supervision for mental health services; however, this supervision is not formal or consistently documented.
- offers structured and regular on-site supervision for mental health services that is focused on staff assessment and/or skill development. This supervision is documented and includes regularly scheduled supervisory periods.

---

seeking safety, or DBT). Supervision is not confused with caseload review or with discussing administrative issues. The focus is dedicated to clinical process.

For example, Betty, a licensed clinical social worker, attended a series of local workshops on CBT for mood and anxiety disorders through the regional Addiction Technology Transfer Center. Betty was able to arrange to be supervised by phone over the course of a year. The agency Betty worked for supported her efforts to acquire these skills since it conceptualized CBT as an evidence-based practice for which its state agency was beginning to require implementation. Betty found that she could use her new skills when supervising other addiction treatment staff members who were called to address a patient's mood or anxiety disorders. Betty used both therapy rating forms (she obtained in the workshop) and audiotape recordings of sessions to help other addiction treatment staff members learn how to perform CBT. Formalizing this supervision process enabled Betty to translate her new skills into practical skill development for staff members. Betty's use of additional time for supervision, beyond the program's previous use of her time to manage administrative concerns and crises, significantly improved the quality of clinical work at her organization.

New research on the supervision process is underway, including the application of motivational interviewing approaches to the supervision process itself.

Evaluate a Mental Health Treatment Program

*In general, a mental health treatment program's **addiction treatment supervision** falls into one of these five categories.*

The program

- lacks the capacity to provide supervision for addiction treatment services.

- provides informal, irregular, and undocumented addiction treatment supervision, usually through an off-site consultant or only in emergent situations on-site.

- offers addiction treatment supervision on-site to staff on a semistructured basis; however, the focus is usually a crisis-management or case-disposition issue.

- offers regular, on-site supervision for addiction treatment services; however, this supervision is not formal or consistently documented.

- offers structured and regular on-site supervision for addiction treatment services that is focused on staff assessment and/or skill development. This supervision is documented and includes regularly scheduled supervisory periods.

Learn More about Clinical Supervision

For more information about the importance of clinical supervision in treatment, read Falender, C. A., & Shafranske, E. P. (2004). *Clinical supervision: A competency-based approach.* Washington, DC: American Psychological Association. Visit www.apa.org/books to purchase the book online.

 See the CD-ROM included with this guidebook for a direct link.

Formal Case Review or Staffings

Has your program established a formal case review process for cases with co-occurring disorders? Since most addiction treatment programs operate using a team approach, there is typically a formal meeting within which new cases are reported, existing cases are periodically reviewed, and soon-to-be-discharged cases are presented. It is also typical that only new cases will be presented in such a meeting. In the case of outpatient programs that essentially operate as a group practice model, perhaps no such group "staff" meetings occur. In addiction treatment programs that offer more enhanced services, not only are these staff meetings more regular in occurrence, they also routinely address the type of psychiatric disorder, its diagnosis, its response to treatment, and the plan for the next level of care. In other words, many addiction treatment programs already review the drug and alcohol use history and symptoms, and discuss the details of the recovery environment and relapse potential. Enhanced addiction treatment programs add to these domains with a systematic focus on psychiatric disorder treatment. More enhanced programs have standard protocols for case review, which are implemented on a consistent basis.

Evaluate Your Formal Case Review or Staffings

It is important to evaluate your program's formal process for reviewing psychiatric and addiction treatment issues in individuals with co-occurring disorders. Your organization's formal review process is used to continually monitor whether the addiction treatment and mental health services being offered are appropriate and effective.

Improve Your Formal Case Review or Staffings

For AOS and MHOS programs to move to the DDC level, the programs must consistently include status reports on patients with co-occurring disorders in case review sessions, staff meetings, or during rounds. Progress with medications, psychiatric issues, substance use, and participation in peer recovery support groups should be included in these discussions in at least a general way.

To move to the DDE level, DDC programs need to record patient progress on psychiatric and addiction treatment in a systematic, consistent fashion. This can be accomplished by having a transcriber in team meetings who records notes on all patient concerns. DDE programs are characterized by routine, systematic, and protocol-driven case review of psychiatric and substance use symptoms. One addiction treatment program uses the Beck Depression Inventory (BDI) and PTSD Checklist scores to ascertain patient status upon admission and again at two-week reviews. All the staff are familiar with the scores of the screening measures used to describe initial psychiatric problem symptom severity. All staff members know the scales on the Mini International Neuropsychiatric Interview (MINI) and the BDI and know how to interpret the clinical importance of scores at the mild, moderate, or severe level. Another residential program lists both psychiatric and substance use problems and designates clinically responsible parties for each disorder. Clinicians then report on patient progress (per treatment plan) at each weekly team meeting. See curriculum ❶ *Screening and Assessment* for patient self-report measures to monitor treatment responses.

On-site Peer Recovery Support

In your program, are on-site peer support persons available for patients with

---

Evaluate an Addiction or Mental Health Treatment Program

*In general, a program's **formal case review or staffings** fall into one of these four categories.*
The program

- does not use a formal review process to review cases of individuals with co-occurring psychiatric disorders and substance use disorders.
- occasionally conducts reviews of co-occurring disorders cases by using an off-site consultant. This is often done informally and is not structured or documented.
- regularly reviews co-occurring disorders cases using an on-site supervisor. There is some minimal documentation that supports the consideration of co-occurring disorders services within this process (e.g., weekly staffings).
- regularly reviews co-occurring disorders cases using a routine, formalized, and consistent protocol. This process is documented and enables the review of targeted interventions for co-occurring disorders cases to determine appropriateness or effectiveness.

co-occurring disorders? This benchmark on peer support overlaps with the treatment and continuity of care benchmarks pertaining to peer recovery supports. Thus, there are three items in total that raise the issue of the availability of peer recovery supports. Peer support is integral to your organization's ability to offer integrated treatment for co-occurring disorders because of its importance in treatment, its ongoing role as support for individuals with chronic disease, and its therapeutic potential for patients by being exposed to another person who can help the patient navigate from the treatment program into the community. This benchmark pertains specifically to access to a person or persons who are peers in recovery.

Historically, many staff members working in addiction treatment programs are also in personal recovery from addiction. The number of staff in recovery from addiction may be lower in outpatient versus residential programs, and even lower when only considering staff members who deliver treatments (versus all employees). Similarly, many staff members working in mental health treatment programs also have personal or family experience with mental health issues.

Personal recovery among staff is no guarantee for the kind of peer recovery support intended by this benchmark. The person that exposes and introduces a patient to peer support can be someone other than an employed staff member. In some programs, the peer recovery support is composed of a group of volunteers who are not employees but have signed privacy forms and meet with some regularity with the program director (who problem solves, clarifies roles, and reiterates boundaries). In other programs, members from a local AA hospital and institution committee (HIC) or "Bridging the Gap" volunteers have been invited to

---

Evaluate an Addiction or Mental Health Treatment Program

*In general, the use of **on-site peer recovery support people** in a program falls into one of these three categories.*

The program

- does not introduce current patients with co-occurring disorders to on-site staff, volunteers, off-site persons, alumni, or peer recovery supports
- consistently introduces current patients to on-site co-occurring disorder peer/alumni supports
- consistently introduces current patients to staff or volunteers on-site who can provide co-occurring disorder peer/alumni support and help individuals transition into peer recovery support groups

do presentations or serve as peer recovery guides. Other recovery-based organizations, such as Friends of Recovery, can also be included in some aspect of formal or informal programming.

Some addiction treatment program leaders become anxious about the prospect of non-staff persons being invited to participate in programming, mostly out of concern for patient confidentiality, but also with trepidation regarding the trustworthiness of the peer supports. These risks can be counterbalanced with potential advantages. It is also possible to be very selective as to who can serve in this capacity and to limit contact to a level that is comfortable for all parties.

Evaluate Your On-site Peer Recovery Support
Ask how your organization is building or plans to build more on-site peer recovery support into your program, with an eye toward introducing patients with co-occurring disorders to a peer mentor.

Improve Your On-site Peer Recovery Support
To move from the AOS or MHOS level to the DDC level, your program must be able to match current patients who have co-occurring disorders with volunteers, alumni, or off-site individuals who have co-occurring disorder histories. The goal is to show a patient who has co-occurring disorders that he or she is not alone and can be successful in connecting with peer recovery support groups.

To move to the DDE level, DDC programs must strategically and routinely make use of alumni, volunteers, and recovering staff to match current patients who have co-occurring disorders with appropriate peers. This can be accomplished by using traditional Twelve Step group mechanisms, HICs, peer-led illness management and recovery groups, staff and volunteer co-led bridge groups, and open alumni and co-occurring disorder meetings. Programs have wrestled with the Health Insurance Portability and Accountability Act (HIPAA), confidentiality, patient safety, and integrity of milieu challenges. Most have agreed these challenges were worth the benefits in facilitating patients' connections to recovering peers. This must occur on-site with a close connection to clinicians and administration.

For example, a hospital was approached by three members of the district AA hospital and institution committee. The members wanted to conduct meetings for the patients at the hospital who had alcohol problems and to hold the meetings in the hospital cafeteria on Friday evenings. The hospital evening intensive outpatient program director, Jim, felt that adding this component to his Monday through Thursday treatment services would be an excellent new feature to his program. Jim agreed to the idea and the meetings have been running for three years. Informally, he has gotten to know some of the "regulars" at the meeting, so he has mentioned to patients who have psychiatric problems to look for Pete, Eddie, or Martha at the Friday-night meetings. Jim bases these "matches" on his awareness of the peer support person's empathy for certain types of people based on personal experience.

•   •   •

Duplicating this page is illegal. Do not copy this material without written permission from the publisher.

133

Workforce: Evaluating Staff Training

Chapter 10 covers training as the final chapter in evaluating how your program's workforce affects your capacity to offer integrated treatment for people with co-occurring disorders.

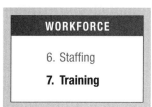

Training utilizes two important benchmarks, both of which are consistent with a realistic and enlightened approach to treatment for persons with co-occurring disorders.

In the sections that follow, the two training benchmarks are defined in detail, and examples of programs that are operating at DDC and DDE levels are given. Suggestions for how a program may consider enhancing its performance on each benchmark are also noted.

Understanding Your Training Practices

Training is often seen as the elixir to all problems or deficiencies in clinical practice. More research from the new field of implementation science continues to demonstrate that training does not change practice. Instead, training may be considered exposure to information, which may result in some change in knowledge, potentially very short-term. But much like you do not expect patients to change from short-term exposures to information, regardless of how accurate or compelling, you should not expect yourself or other clinicians to change so rapidly. Instead, more realistically, you might consider training as the first step, or perhaps second step, in a systematic plan to change practice or protocol. The step before training may actually be deciding what practice you want to implement and then figuring out how you are going to sustain it—even before you train staff in it.

Working Knowledge

What types of working knowledge (training and skills) on assessment and treatment of co-occurring disorders do staff members have? Some exposure to basic information about co-occurring disorders is essential. Basic information may include addressing addiction treatment staff members' concerns about

> **TRAINING BENCHMARKS**
>
> Training encompasses two benchmarks that should be evaluated in this order:
>
> 1. Working knowledge
>
> 2. Cross-training of staff

stigma, potential dangerousness to others or self, safety, the meaning of psychiatric symptoms, and some general descriptions about the types of disorders. This basic training segment may entail a self-assessment of attitudes and stereotypes, as well as some awareness-raising about the prevalence or expected rates of the most common disorders (mood, anxiety, and so forth). Lastly, a basic training may also involve some preliminary information about screening and referral.

Staff may need to know how to quickly assess for the likelihood of common disorders (such as by using standardized screening measures) and for the key indicators of acuity (suicidality, dangerousness, impulsivity, capacity for self-care, and self-harm potential). In as much as a treatment agency supports staff training, either by annual allocation of funds per staff member or in paid time off, training in co-occurring disorders should be strategic. For example, several agency directors mandate that 25 percent of paid staff training be in the area of ethics. Having the same level of strategy for co-occurring disorders training is recommended in addiction and mental health treatment programs.

Evaluate Your Working Knowledge

In thinking about the overall level of knowledge your staff may have, you might review the program's requirements for basic skills and training with regard to co-occurring disorders as well as strategic training plans. Determine if staff members meet these requirements. Specifically, assess if staff have training in the prevalence of co-occurring disorders, the screening and assessment of co-occurring disorders, the signs and symptoms of co-occurring disorders, and in triage and treatment decision making.

Improve Your Working Knowledge

Although training is the customary means of imparting information, it may not be sufficient in yielding practice change. For AOS and MHOS programs to move to the DDC level, the programs must strategically train the majority of staff in basic co-occurring disorders issues including attitudes, prevalence, screening, triage, and brief intervention. These trainings may be strategically directed using the existing training budget or release time and incorporated into a training plan. As an example of how to incorporate training into existing structures, one program in the Midwest provides nine in-service training sessions and has committed one-third of these sessions to co-occurring disorders. The training program includes all staff, from clinical supervisors and residential aides to front office administrative support staff.

To move to the DDE level, DDC programs must train all staff in basic co-occurring disorder issues. The program must also train designated staff in more advanced issues—including differential diagnostics, evidence-based pharmacological and psychosocial practices, and principles of preferred or evidenced-based practices—and in learning specific new treatments for adaptation for persons with co-occurring disorders. Much like administrators in DDC programs, administrators in DDE programs strategically direct staff training and incorporate the cost of doing so into existing allocations wherever possible.

Cross-Training of Staff

Are clinical staff members cross-trained in mental health and substance use disorders, including both pharmacotherapies and psychosocial treatment? This benchmark covers the need for certain staff members—particularly those providing direct service—to be more integrated at the clinician level. Recall that treatment

---

Evaluate an Addiction or Mental Health Treatment Program

*In general, the **working knowledge** of a program's staff will fall into one of these following five categories.*

The program

- does not require staff to be trained on basic co-occurring disorder issues and symptoms. The staff has no training.

- includes some staff with basic knowledge of co-occurring disorders. Staff members are encouraged to attend training, but it is not part of the program's overall strategic plan.

- requires staff to have basic training on co-occurring disorders. The majority of the program staff is trained on co-occurring disorder issues, including the prevalence of co-occurring disorders, screening and assessment of co-occurring disorders, the signs and symptoms of co-occurring disorders, and triage and treatment decision making for co-occurring disorders.

- requires staff to have basic training in co-occurring disorder issues and also has staff trained in advanced co-occurring disorder issues and specifically targeted treatments. However, this is not part of the program's overall strategic plan.

- requires all staff to have basic training in co-occurring disorder issues and some designated staff to have advanced training as outlined in the program's strategic plan.

services could be integrated at the system level, the program level, or the individual clinician level. This benchmark seeks to assess the degree to which the program has developed clinicians at the integrated level. At this juncture, this benchmark does not precisely define "cross-trained" or "expertise." Licensure or certification refers to expertise, but in some cases expertise may be evident without formal licensure or certification.

More enhanced treatment programs have developed a group of clinicians who possess both mental health and addiction expertise. Psychiatric physicians may have additional certification in addiction psychiatry or addiction medicine, and clinical psychologists may have advanced certification in psychoactive substance use disorders through the American Psychological Association. Social workers may also have additional special qualifications, and mental health counselors and addiction counselors may have dual licensure. As stated previously, there are several initiatives by states (e.g., Pennsylvania and Connecticut) for certification in co-occurring disorders. At this time, no agreed-upon core curriculum for this type of certification or for basic or advanced training exists.

This benchmark item would be understood as more advanced training and expertise than discussed in the previous benchmark. Clinicians at this level should have already completed some "basic" training in co-occurring disorders and have a firm grasp on attitudes and stigma, prevalence, screening and assessment,

---

Evaluate an Addiction or Mental Health Treatment Program

In general, a program falls into one of these five categories.

The program
- does not cross-train staff in co-occurring disorder interventions and does not have plans to do so.
- has less than half of the staff cross-trained in co-occurring disorder interventions. Cross-training is not necessarily included in the overall training plan for program staff.
- has more than half of the staff cross-trained in co-occurring disorder interventions. Cross-training is part of the overall training plan for the program staff but is not fully implemented.
- has nearly all (75 percent) of the staff cross-trained in co-occurring disorder interventions. Cross-training is part of the overall training plan for the program staff but is not fully implemented.
- has all staff members cross-trained in co-occurring disorder interventions. Cross-training is part of the overall training plan for the program staff and has been largely implemented.

differential diagnosis, and treatment planning. Clinicians at this level are more at the cusp of learning to deliver interventions, whether psychosocial or medication, specifically designed for patients with co-occurring disorders. Clinicians at this level would be capable of delivering, with competence and adherence, the therapies outlined in curricula ❷, ❸, and ❺.

Evaluate Your Cross-Training of Staff

In analyzing this benchmark, review your program's strategic training plan including the definition and use of "cross-training" in mental health and substance use disorders. In addition, identify the number of clinicians who have completed cross-training and determine if this type of training is supported in your program. Are clinicians capable of delivering specialized interventions to persons with co-occurring disorders?

Improve Your Cross-Training of Staff

For AOS and MHOS programs to move to the DDC level, the programs must cross-train a portion of staff in both addiction and mental health treatments. This should be done in at least a somewhat-consistent fashion. The goal is for 50 percent to 75 percent of the staff to be cross-trained. To move to the DDE level, all front-line clinical staff need to be cross-trained so they can all handle patients with co-occurring disorders. For programs to be at the DDE level, 90 percent of the staff should be cross-trained.

● ● ●

Balancing Organizational Resources with Needs

Chapters 4 to 10 of this guide have covered the seven key dimensions of the DDCAT index:

▶ **Dimension 1: Program Structure**

Does your overall program structure help or inhibit providing services for individuals with co-occurring disorders?

▶ **Dimension 2: Program Milieu**

What is the "culture" of your program? Are the staff and physical environment welcoming and receptive to individuals with co-occurring disorders?

▶ **Dimensions 3 and 4: Clinical Process**

How do your clinical assessment and treatment procedures and protocols rate in relation to co-occurring disorder assessment and treatment?

▶ **Dimension 5: Continuity of Care**

How does your program handle long-term treatment for individuals with co-occurring disorders? Do monitoring, care, and peer support transition beyond treatment?

▶ **Dimension 6: Staffing**

Are any staff members capable and willing to assess and treat individuals with co-occurring disorders? What are the hiring patterns of your program and long-term goals for hiring in regard to expertise in co-occurring disorders?

▶ **Dimension 7: Training**

Does your program provide strategic staff training and support for the assessment and treatment of individuals with co-occurring disorders?

After reading this material, some addiction treatment or mental health agencies will make a conscious decision to achieve either the DDC- or DDE-level status on every benchmark within each dimension, which will put them in a position to provide excellent services to people with co-occurring disorders. Either through utilization of existing funding, grant support, or as an investment, these treatment providers may not see resources as an obstacle. For these addiction

141

treatment or mental health organizations, the organization's mission will be to implement the most effective services for patients with co-occurring disorders—no matter how challenging the process.

Understanding Cost Barriers

Most addiction treatment and mental health agencies will not be able to take all the steps they would like to enhance their treatment services. Choices will need to be made. As stated previously, some of the benchmark items have costs attached to them, whereas others do not. The following scale gives the potential range in costs for implementation.

$	No Cost	$0 to less than $100
$$	Low Cost	$100 to $10,000
$$$	Moderate Cost	between $10,000 and $40,000
$$$$	High Cost	more than $40,000

The most significant costs to implement change to increase capacity for treating co-occurring disorders would be in hiring and/or increasing the number of hours for physicians or prescribers. The estimates include the potential for a contractual or consulting relationship with a prescriber for a significant block of time (one or more full days per week). The presence of this person would leverage at least three benchmarks.

Cost of Policy Changes

Changes in program policy that would affect licensure and certification, as well as financial processes, may also be cost-driven. The application costs for these certifications and licenses vary by state. The up-front cost to prepare materials and make programmatic changes (such as in policy and procedure manuals and staff credentials) is generally less than the license or certificate itself.

Cost of Staff Changes

Other higher cost changes would include the clinical and staffing changes necessary to support an increase in the range of acceptance of patients for treatment with less regard for acuity. This may involve the capacity to manage more acute psychiatric or substance-related states and having more staff on hand to observe, supervise, and treat patients. Qualified nursing personnel may be needed. Programs may also need to consider alterations to the physical settings.

FIGURE 8

Benchmark Item and Estimated Cost Range

BENCHMARK ITEM	ESTIMATED COST RANGE
Program structure	
Mission statement	$$
Licensure/certification	$$$
Relationship with mental health service provider	$$
Financial incentives	$$
Program milieu	
Social environment	$
Physical environment	$
Assessment	
Standardized screening	$
Routine assessment	$
Routine diagnosis	$
Psychiatric and substance use history	$
Acceptance based on acuity	$$$$
Acceptance based on severity	$$
Stage-wise assessment	$
Treatment	
Routine treatment plans	$
Monitor both disorders	$
Procedures for psychiatric emergencies	$
Stage-wise treatment	$$
Medication management	$$$$
Psychosocial treatments	$$
Patient education	$
Family education and support	$
Facilitation to peer recovery support groups	$
Continuity of care	
Discharge plan	$
Capacity to maintain continuity	$$
Co-occurring recovery focus	$
Connection to peer support in community	$
Medication continuity	$$$$
Staffing	
Physician or prescriber	$$$$
Mental health license or expertise	$$$
Clinical supervision	$$
Case review	$
Peer recovery mentors	$
Training	
Basic	$
Cross-training/advanced	$$$

Identifying the Program Level You Would Like to Achieve

Improving your performance on some benchmarks may involve some cost to hire and or support clinicians to become mental health or addiction licensed or certified. The majority of changes or enhancements can be implemented with very little financial cost. The cost becomes more so a matter of motivation, time, and the effort to change direction.

Given this fact, the changes or enhancements that any program intends to make may not be as resource-driven or limited as one might think. The task instead becomes deciding, preferably through consensus across stakeholders associated with the program, what changes are desired and who is responsible for seeing them through.

This process of organizational change, outlined more fully in the next chapter, is not one to enter into without a right hand filled with focus and a left hand filled with patience.

Some experts have suggested that, given the high prevalence rate of psychiatric disorders in addiction treatment and the high rates of substance use disorders in mental health treatment settings, all programs should at least be DDC. Some costs will likely be associated with movement from an AOS- (or MHOS-) to a DDC-level program. There also may be some agency directors who want to strive for the highest level of dual diagnosis capability, DDE, and even more cost will likely be associated with movement from DDC- to DDE-level services. Research is presently underway to examine the costs to programs who have made these changes, though at this time these data are not available.

Many states and providers are voluntarily seeking to achieve a DDC-level status at minimum. On the horizon in certain states may be a requirement that states are at least DDC in order to maintain level funding. Other states may incentivize DDC and DDE programs, while holding AOS and MHOS programs at level funding. Since no new monies are typically available for addiction or mental health services, it is unclear how this latter fiscal policy might be accomplished.

Much like the fact that not all community hospital emergency rooms are level one trauma centers, not all addiction or mental health treatment programs will likely ever be or need to be DDE. A rational model suggests that a certain number of programs should be DDE, however. What this portion is—such as the number of beds or outpatient slots per 100,000 people in a given population—has not yet been determined. Thus every community and every provider must make their own assessment of need and of available resources for AOS, MHOS, DDC, or DDE services. This local approach will likely override any estimates made from a public health-oriented calculation.

Not all persons with substance use disorders have psychiatric disorders. Not all persons with mental health disorders have problems with drugs or alcohol. Some persons are in stable recovery from both disorders and may prefer to be in treatment in more traditional AOS or MHOS programs. Therefore, it is likely that these programs will have a future, particularly in a residential level of care format, or in programs that offer long-term environmental (housing, social) support for persons in more sustained recovery.

•   •   •

Duplicating this page is illegal. Do not copy this material without written permission from the publisher.

145

CHAPTER 12

Program Assessment and Change Initiatives

Understanding the General Principles of Program Change

The emerging field of implementation science is slowly informing us about how the process of organizational, systems, program, and practice change takes place. Likewise, it is also advising us on the best ways to change effectively. *The Change Book,* published by the Addiction Technology Transfer Center Network, provided the field with some early insights on this process, drawn heavily from the work of Everett Rogers's *Diffusion of Innovations.* Rogers observed that there are different types of adopters, and innovations of all types are embraced and utilized at varying paces and over time.

Data is just beginning to be collected about program and systems changes associated with enhancements of program services for patients with co-occurring disorders. As these data are analyzed and there is the opportunity for more systematic observations, better information will become available.

Meanwhile, there seem to be several key steps in the process of program change.

The Seven Key Steps of Program Change

1. The first step is a decision made by key leadership. A person at the top of the organization, who could be an agency director, a program director, a medical director, a respected physician, or a key clinical opinion leader makes a case to the organization that changes are needed.

2. The next step (which also could come first but must be fully supported by the person in step one) involves the development of a reasonable consensus among key stakeholders that this change should take place. The key stakeholders might consist of the key leadership described in step one, but also can include frontline clinicians, the community partners (referral sources and associated providers), and consumers.

3. The third step involves becoming organized about the change. This involves getting as specific as possible about what needs to change, how the change will take place, who will be responsible for it, and how key stakeholders will know if it is working. One approach that has worked at this stage is the formation of a "steering committee" within the program. These people

Duplicating this page is illegal. Do not copy this material without written permission from the publisher.

147

will meet regularly and make a commitment to the change and to one another to increase organizational accountability for planned action steps.

4. Step four often involves developing a concrete plan.

5. Step five is where individual staff members begin to actualize the planned changes. Typically this involves delegating and performing specific tasks as directed by the steering committee.

6. Step six involves the process of deciding if the change was worthwhile. Are the stakeholders and the steering committee happy with it? Did it accomplish all that they wanted it to?

7. Step seven involves sustainability. If the answers to the two questions in step six were affirmative, then step seven asks, "How does the program maintain the change?" Sustainability is particularly important if the change was financially supported for a short term (by a special grant or a research study or hinges entirely on the presence of one or two people). How would the change fare if this person left? What will happen after the grant money runs out? Sustainability will be more challenging with short-term funding than with long-term funding, such as with a long-term grant or by a commitment to use an ongoing portion of organizational revenue as funding.

Identifying Your Organizational Readiness to Change

Much like the stages of change model for patients, organizations and programs can be placed along the continuum of readiness from precontemplation to contemplation to action to maintenance. With simple self-assessments/ surveys, clinicians'

Measure Organizational Readiness

A measure of organizational readiness for change (ORC) was developed by Wayne Lehman and colleagues at the Institute of Behavioral Research at Texas Christian University. The ORC is a self-assessment that can be completed by agency administrators and/or clinical staff and assesses the organizational context within which change efforts might be focused. The ORC contains several subscales including communication, physical environment, stability, and cohesiveness as examples of factors that might influence organizational readiness for adopting new practices. The ORC is available without charge at www.ibr.tcu.edu.

See the CD-ROM included with this guidebook for a direct link to this resource.

readiness to adopt evidence-based practices in addiction can be easily placed on this continuum. Organizations are more difficult to assess for readiness because there may be differing perspectives among agency leadership, key clinical supervisors, and frontline clinicians.

Initiating Program Change

The seven steps previously outlined may be useful as a general process for approaching organizational changes to support integrated treatment services for patients with co-occurring disorders as outlined in this *Clinical Administrator's Guidebook.*

If you are a key leader in your organization or treatment program, you may want to present this *Clinical Administrator's Guidebook* to other leaders in your organization who can help champion and lead your program through the suggested process of forming a steering committee. This committee will need to become familiar with the benchmarks listed in chapters 4 to 10 of this guidebook, and perhaps make a priority list ranked according to the changes most desired, or perhaps even more pragmatic—create a list based on ease of achievability.

This will not only be practical, but it will begin to build some momentum for the change process. It is always good to start out with a success and take it from there. A sense of efficacy and possibility can quickly result. Since most organizations have tried multiple times to change without success, and most have watched many initiatives come and go, an early experience with success is critically important.

After reviewing this *Clinical Administrator's Guidebook* with your steering committee and rank-ordering the benchmarks to address, you can begin by making a list of specific change objectives. This guidebook provides practical, specific guidance on how to make changes on each benchmark objective.

Utilizing the DDCAT Methodology

After reading this *Clinical Administrator's Guidebook* and following the practical guidance on each benchmark, you may already have an excellent idea about your program's current ability to offer integrated treatment for co-occurring disorders. On the other hand, there is no substitute for the objective, unbiased assessment you can obtain when using an outside professional to score your program using the DDCAT Index.

Obtain the DDCAT Index (or DDCMHT), scoring component, and Excel scoring workbook from the Dartmouth Psychiatric Research Center Web site at http://dms.dartmouth.edu/prc/dual/atsr. See the CD-ROM included with this guidebook for links to these items.

Let us assume that you have completed the DDCAT (or DDCMHT) assessment and have recorded your observations or ratings in the DDCAT Excel scoring workbook. The next step is to look at your program's DDCAT/DDCMHT profile.

Understanding Your Program's DDCAT/DDCMHT Profile

At the end of the DDCAT assessment, you will receive a DDCAT profile via the Excel workbook. This profile depicts your program's scores relative to the AOS, DDC, and DDE criteria overall. On the DDCMHT profile, MHOS-level scores will be used. It also rates your performance for each of the seven DDCAT dimensions.

THE SEVEN KEY DIMENSIONS OF THE DDCAT AND DDCMHT INDEX

Dimension 1 . . . . Program structure

Dimension 2 . . . . Program milieu

Dimensions 3 and 4 . . . Clinical process

Dimension 5 . . . . Continuity of care

Dimension 6 . . . . Staffing

Dimension 7 . . . . Training

You may choose to interpret your DDCAT profile by identifying dimensions you feel reflect your best work. You may also choose to focus on improving low-scoring dimensions that may indicate areas for quality improvement initiatives. Some of these dimensions—for example, program structure or staffing—may involve an extra cost to address. Other dimensions—for example, training or assessment—involve few, if any, costs to implement. Once you examine your profile, you can identify the specific dimensions you wish to address in order to improve your program's ability to offer integrated treatment for co-occurring disorders.

Understanding Your Program's DDCAT/DDCMHT Interpretation, Feedback, and Reports

The conduct and scoring of the DDCAT will produce scores that categorize your program as AOS, DDC, or DDE within each of the seven dimensions. The DDCMHT will produce scores that categorize your program as MHOS, DDC, or DDE.

Since details of the measures are still in progress, programs are urged not to make too much of the AOS or MHOS, DDC, or DDE categorization option. However, many will insist on using the labels as a simple way to define their program's capacity to offer integrated treatment to people with co-occurring disorders.

Your program's DDCAT (or DDCMHT) dimension scores are the average scores of all the benchmark items listed within each dimension. The scores on these dimensions can be examined for relative highs and lows, and may be connected with the agency's own readiness to address specific, if not all, areas. These averages can also be depicted on a chart (line graph) which is an easy visual aid that shows where your program falls (above or below midline) on each benchmark. These charts can be used in PowerPoint or other presentations to inform program leadership of the dimensions that are strengths and to note areas for potential improvement. As you reassess your program at intervals you specify, the charts can be used for an easy visual comparison to indicate how your program is changing over time. This is a great way to document your continuous quality improvement for each benchmark.

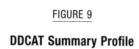

FIGURE 9

DDCAT Summary Profile

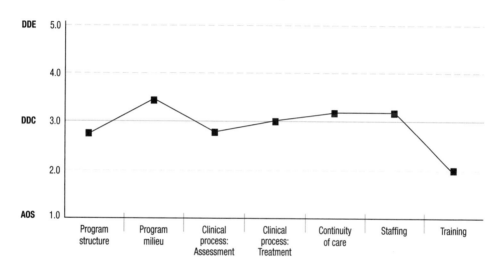

Figure 9 represents an example of a DDCAT assessment profile of an addiction treatment program that is at or above the DDC level on program milieu, treatment, continuity of care, and staffing. This is a program where a patient can talk about his or her psychiatric disorder and be attended to by qualified staff with mental

The Excel program file for the DDCAT that is used to score, record, and summarize your program's itemized ratings is available from the Dartmouth Web site (www.dartmouth.edu).

A link to this file is on the CD-ROM included with this guidebook in the "DDCAT Resources" document.

This Excel program also generates a graphic image that represents your program's performance in each of the seven DDCAT dimensions.

health expertise who use adaptations of best practices for patients with substance use disorders. An obvious area of potential challenge for this program is in the area of training. The training dimension might suggest that although qualified, this program's staff could benefit from education that focuses on specific practices for patients with co-occurring disorders (rather than loose adaptations of existing practices). It would seem that this program would be relatively receptive to this type of program change, and that given its relative strengths on most dimensions, the practice would have a good chance of success.

• • •

Continuous Quality Improvements and Process Improvement Strategies

CHAPTER 13

Understanding the Use of the DDCAT for Continuous Quality Improvement

You may want to use this *Clinical Administrator's Guidebook* along with the DDCAT Toolkit—a link to the toolkit is located in the "DDCAT Resources" file on the CD-ROM that accompanies this guidebook—to plan and measure the outcome of continuous quality improvement activities in your program.

Establishing Program Goals

Program goals can range from changing your mission statement (dimension 1, benchmark 1), to more carefully supervising and reviewing treatment plans for a co-occurring disorder focus (dimension 4, benchmark 1), to increasing the time your medical director has to attend treatment team meetings (dimension 6, benchmark 1). The timeline for goal implementation can range, but sometimes it's helpful to start by identifying and staging plans based on ease of implementation (taking care of easy improvements first).

Three Steps to Use the DDCAT for Continuous Quality Improvement

1. First, assess your program's current capabilities using the *Clinical Administrator's Guidebook* and the DDCAT Index to obtain a "baseline" assessment of your program.

2. After reviewing your DDCAT scores, develop change plans that include goals, objectives, interventions, responsible persons, and projected target dates that address each benchmark where program improvement is needed. This *Clinical Administrator's Guidebook* and the DDCAT Toolkit can support this process.

3. After you succeed in getting your program to the level you seek, direct your efforts at sustaining your improved capacity to serve people with co-occurring disorders.

For example, you can begin to review all your treatment plans now (by the end of the month), then propose a new mission statement by the next board meeting (in the next three months), and plan to expand your medical director's hours (in the next six months). Your executive director may choose to work with the board on developing the mission statement, the clinical director could work with the three clinical supervisors to review the counselors' treatment plans, and the administrator will begin the process to expand the hours of the medical director.

Figure 10 demonstrates a sample implementation plan that specifies program goals, objectives, action required, responsible parties, target date, and measurable outcome. See the CD-ROM included with this guidebook for a blank, reproducible copy of this worksheet.

Defining Program Change

There are many changes that can be made within each benchmark to improve your capacity to serve people with co-occurring disorders. These changes generally fall into four categories: policy, protocol, staff training, and clinical practice.

Target areas for program change include

1. Changes in policy: internal policy changes, policy changes with regard to community partners, or state or regional policy changes

2. Changes in protocol: changes involving screening, assessment, and treatment of patients with co-occurring disorders

---

Six Steps to Actualize Program Goals

1. Identify the DDCAT (or DDCMHT) dimension you would like to improve. This is your goal.

2. Identify the specific DDCAT (or DDCMHT) benchmark items you seek to improve. This is your list of objectives.

3. Identify the action that needs to occur to improve your performance on each benchmark item.

4. Identify the person responsible for the execution of each action item you listed in step three.

5. Identify target dates for each action item you listed in step three.

6. Identify measurable outcomes that match the action items listed in step three and the goal listed in step one.

FIGURE 10

Sample Implementation Plan Using This Guidebook and DDCAT Dimensions

GOAL (DDCAT DIMENSION)	OBJECTIVE (DDCAT BENCHMARK ITEM)	INTERVENTION	RESPONSIBILITY	TIME FRAME	MEASURABLE OUTCOME
I. Program structure	I. Mission statement	Revise mission statement with co-occurring disorder focus	Deputy director	2 months	Put the new mission statement in brochures
	III. Relationship with local community mental health (MH) center	Develop charter agreement with Blaine MH center	Deputy director	1 month	Signed charter agreement with Blaine MH center
II. Program milieu	II. Materials for psychiatric problems in waiting areas and for patient handouts	Obtain from NIMH Web site for copying and distribution	Clinical director (will delegate to administrative assistant)	1 month	Put materials in racks and psychiatric information in select patient workbooks
III. Assessment	VII. Stage-wise assessment	Obtain form from curriculum ❶ *Screening and Assessment;* put this form in all new charts; supervise counselors' use of this form	Intensive outpatient (IOP) program director	1 month	Put this form in all new admits' charts
IV. Treatment	IX. Specialized groups for psychiatric disorders	Use curriculum ❷ *Integrating Combined Therapies* and begin weekly groups for all patients in IOP treatment, then in residential treatment	IOP and residential clinical supervisors; supervised by the clinical director and program directors	4 months	1 group started in IOP and 1 in residential: once a week
V. Continuity of care	I. Discharge plans	Supervise and monitor all plans	Clinical directors	1 month	Plans address both psychiatric and substance use disorders. 80 percent of plans at 1 month; 100 percent of plans at 3 months
VI. Staffing	III. Supervision	Supervise new groups using curriculum ❷ *Integrating Combined Therapies*	Clinical supervisors	4 months	Supervise weekly 1-on-1 happening
VII. Training	II. Cross-training/advanced training	Send 1 supervisor and 2 staff members from IOP and residential to training for curriculum ❷ *Integrating Combined Therapies*	Clinical supervisors and volunteer clinicians	3 months	Attend and complete training and get all materials

3. Changes in staff training: improvements in the attitudes, knowledge base, and experience of staff

4. Changes in clinical practice: improvements in supervision of staff, support for staff, and staff awareness that patients are improving

In dimension 1 (program structure), changes in policy are the most effective interventions, and these are typically best undertaken by senior leadership. For changes in dimension 2 (program milieu), dimension 3 (clinical practice: assessment and clinical practice: treatment), and dimension 4 (continuity of care), the best interventions are changes in protocol. These changes in protocol typically involve new procedures that after a period of some training are monitored and supervised by key clinical leaders or clinical supervisors. These may be as simple as developing and implementing standard screening forms, assessment protocols, or treatment plan forms.

Initiating Program Change

Program change can be challenging to initiate and sustain in even the most willing and well-intentioned context. Use the implementation worksheet (included on the CD-ROM that accompanies this guidebook) to plan and execute your goals. Share this document with your steering committee members to galvanize them toward a common objective. When you fill out the implementation worksheet, it helps to designate explicit, concrete objectives along with measurable outcomes. This eliminates the amorphous nature of most change initiatives. Some programs construct their implementation forms with the utmost attention to specific DDCAT scores. For example, if the program scored at a two on a particular DDCAT benchmark, the measurable goal may be to score a three on the next DDCAT assessment. Although this is an understandable application of the practical aspect of the DDCAT and its clear anchors for scoring, it also has the potential to confuse the "test" with the "skill." For this reason, if DDCAT (or DDCMHT) scores are used as objectives, they are best paired with observable changes in practice or protocol.

Measuring Program Change

The DDCAT (or DDCMHT for mental health treatment programs) can provide an addiction treatment program with a practical blueprint and the tools necessary to achieve an increased capacity to treat people with co-occurring disorders. Since the DDCAT and DDCMHT can be readministered at different intervals of time, they can also be used to measure your program's ability to execute and sustain changes over time.

Once your defined changes are implemented, you will notice that improvements in your program's DDCAT or DDCMHT scores are directly related to improvements in your program's treatment outcomes for patients.

Understanding Process Improvement Strategies

Process improvement strategies are strategies that have been created and disseminated through the Network for the Improvement of Addiction Treatment (NIATx) initiative funded by the Robert Wood Johnson Foundation. These typically involve very basic practice improvement strategies such as reducing the amount of time patients wait on the phone for assessment, the time between the patient's first call and appointment, and the time between assessment and initiation of treatment. Measures might include changes on these specific program indicators but also changes in show rates (the percent of people who call and who present for services; i.e., the percent of patients who keep appointments) and treatment engagement. How would these measures pertain to co-occurring disorders? Simple measures of process improvement might be gathered before any attempt to implement aspects of this *Clinical Administrator's Guidebook* are undertaken. For example, first you may want to develop a way to identify persons with co-occurring disorders (for instance, by using information you gathered from phone screens regarding patients' prior mental health treatment, current medications, and ability to verbalize a mental health diagnosis). Count the number of people of all inquiries who meet your criteria for a co-occurring disorder diagnosis and schedule appointments. Count these people and compare the number to all appointments that are kept. Track patient engagement (attendance at two sessions within the first month for outpatients, completing one week for those in residential programs). Do these rates of engagement show change as a result of implementing recommendations from this *Clinical Administrator's Guidebook?* In other words, has your front door access for persons with co-occurring disorders improved? Once the patients are in the door, do they decide to stay?

Measuring Changes in Treatment Outcomes

Reliable indicators of improved treatment outcomes for patients—from baseline, to post-treatment, and over time—are often difficult and expensive for most programs to gather and study. Programs with the capability to gather and study such data are encouraged to do so to document how changes in policy, practice, and workforce translate to improvements in patients' lives.

NIATx

The Network for the Improvement of Addiction Treatment (NIATx) is a partnership of addiction treatment services researchers, community treatment providers, recovering persons, and human factors engineers who have been developing practical means of improving the quality of routine health care. Included in these efforts are pragmatic approaches to "customer service" such as improving intake call response, reducing wait time to first appointment, reducing time to admission, and utilizing walk-thru approaches to learn about the experience of treatment (see next page). In addition, the findings of the NIATx group have strongly reinforced the importance of the use of data to guide program level decision making. Recent reports from the NIATx group (e.g., McCarty et al., 2007) describe the application of treatment quality indicators such as access, engagement, and retention.

These "NIATx indicators" can serve as proxies for patient outcomes, and a clinical program administrator can track changes in these indicators as quality improvement strategies are implemented for persons with co-occurring disorders. As any treatment program moves from the AOS or MHOS level to the DDC or DDE levels, these changes should translate to measurable changes in the NIATx indicators. For more information about NIATx, visit www.niatx.net.

Washington Circle Indicators

The Washington Circle indicators are precursors to the NIATx project and focus on engagement, retention, and linkage indicators. So, coupled with the NIATx

---

Gathering Patient Outcomes

A few methods of gathering patient outcomes include

1. NIATx

2. Washington Circle indicators

3. Walk-thru methodologies

4. Management information system data

5. Patient satisfaction surveys

These methods are readily available and affordable to the majority of addiction treatment and mental health providers.

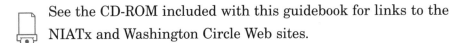 See the CD-ROM included with this guidebook for links to the NIATx and Washington Circle Web sites.

---

indicators for engagement, an addiction treatment program, such as a residential detoxification or rehabilitation program, may also study successful linkage with outpatient services. The benchmark indicator would be the percent of patients who attend the outpatient session off-site within one or two weeks from discharge/ transfer. This outcome measure would also have to begin with trying to identify patients with co-occurring disorders (as perhaps identified on the assessment, diagnosis, treatment plan, or discharge form). In addition, it would involve comparing the number of patients with co-occurring disorders versus those without co-occuring disorders who attend outpatient services after discharge/transfer, before and after the implementation of the benchmark suggestions in this *Clinical Administrator's Guidebook.*

Walk-thru Methodologies

Somewhat related to the work of NIATx is the resurrection of the walk-thru methodology to learn about the process of entry and treatment into services from the patient's point of view. Typically, this method involves the use of a "stooge" or actor pretending to be a person with a co-occurring disorder. First, this person may report problems with drugs or alcohol and then reveal some psychiatric symptoms. How are these problems dealt with by the person who answers the phone and takes the necessary information for the initial assessment? If the walk-thru process continues and the stooge in fact gets an appointment, how does this appointment go? Does the person feel welcomed, stigmatized, rejected, or accepted? Typically, the walk-thru methods focus on the front end of treatment and are an excellent means to assess access issues, and an effective and dramatic way to assess the culture of a program.

Management Information System Data

States and comprehensive programs often, but not always, collect aggregate data for billing and financial services. These data may also include some clinically descriptive data such as diagnosis, type of discharge, and length of stay. If these data can be grouped by diagnosis, and diagnoses for both mental health and substance use disorders are recorded, it may be possible to monitor admission trends (percent and type of admissions with co-occurring disorders), treatment completion, and length of stay. Examine data of those with versus those without co-occurring disorders before and after the implementation of the benchmark suggestions in this *Clinical Administrator's Guidebook.*

If diagnostic information is available, it may also be possible to group admissions by quadrant. (See the article entitled "Assessing the Dual Diagnosis Capability of Addiction Treatment Services" by McGovern, Matzkin, & Giard for this methodology. The article is located on the CD-ROM included with this guidebook. Changes in percent of admissions by quadrant would also be an important indicator of changes in services and outcomes for patients with co-occurring disorders.

Patient Satisfaction Surveys

Many programs, whether by choice or mandate, collect patient satisfaction information. These surveys, ranging in item count from two to thirty questions, often are good indicators of overall comfort with services received. Most studies have found satisfaction to be extremely high, but typically only satisfied patients elect to complete the surveys. Nonetheless, for programs that collect this information, it may be possible to identify persons with co-occurring disorders before and after the implementation of changes and discern if patient satisfaction has in any way shifted favorably.

• • •

▼

CONCLUSION

LETTER FROM THE AUTHORS

Our primary purpose in creating the Co-occurring Disorders Program was to help people with co-occurring psychiatric and substance use disorders improve their chances for recovery. Our objective in this *Clinical Administrator's Guidebook* was to assist providers in developing services that are evidence-based, which will likely improve outcomes for patients with co-occurring disorders. We developed this component with practicality in mind so that it could be readily translated by an agency or program into policy, practice, and workforce changes. In addition, we attempted to appreciate the complexity and relative poverty associated with real-world conditions on the front lines of mental health and addiction treatment services. We strove to make things as simple and economic as possible. We provided as many materials as we could for free. When possible, we offered directions to free resources that are in the public domain. We also recognized the challenges in work-force improvements, in terms of adequate compensation, recruitment of new staff, and turnover of existing staff. We believe the processes of skill augmentation, clinical supervision, quality case review, and increasing clinical efficacy recommended in this program will be attractive to your program staff. Nonetheless, it is hard to compete for a workforce when often staff can receive better compensation in jobs half as demanding. On the other hand, those working in the addiction or mental health field typically rate personal fulfillment more highly than economic gain. We hope these values remain intact.

The Co-occurring Disorders Program is a first edition. We expect the evidence-base of this program to provide us with more knowledge about what works for various types of treatment providers, and what factors in this program are more important than others. We have provided you, the reader, with what we know thus far. We hope to update this information with new evidence, with information from exciting research that is presently underway, with feedback from many of our colleagues who use the DDCAT and its associated materials across the United States and internationally, and with information from those of you who apply the benchmarks in this *Clinical Administrator's Guidebook* to your treatment programs. We hope you offer us feedback on what worked and what did not in your program.

Please utilize the resources found in each of the components that make up the Co-occurring Disorders Program. Taken as a whole, this program should provide you with the structure and content to enable you to offer the best treatment services available for people with co-occurring disorders. Please use not only the clinician's guides included in the program, but also the program DVD, *A Guide for Living with Co-occurring Disorders.* This DVD can serve as a vehicle to educate patients and families to improve patient outcomes; in turn, these stakeholders can educate policymakers and providers about what each patient needs to recover a life worth living.

• • •

▼

RESOURCES

References

American Psychiatric Association (2000). *Diagnostic and statistical manual of mental disorders* (4th ed., text revision). Washington, DC: American Psychiatric Association.

American Society of Addiction Medicine. (2001). *ASAM patient placement criteria for the treatment of substance-related disorders* (2nd ed.–revised). Chevy Chase, MD: American Society of Addiction Medicine, Inc.

Brady, K. T., Dansky, B. S., Back, S. E., Foa, E. B., & Carroll, K. M. (2001). Exposure therapy in the treatment of PTSD among cocaine-dependent individuals: Preliminary findings. *Journal of Substance Abuse Treatment, 21,* 47–54.

Brown, R. A., & Ramsey, S. E. (2000). Addressing comorbid depressive symptomatology in alcohol treatment. *Professional Psychology: Research and Practice, 31*(4), 418–422.

Gotham, H. J., Brown, J. L., Comaty, J., & McGovern, M. P. (2008). *The Dual Diagnosis Capability in Mental Health Treatment (DDCMHT) Index.* (Version 3.2). Kansas City, MO: Mid-America Addiction Technology Transfer Center.

Hien, D. A., Cohen, L. R., Miele, G. M., Litt, L. C., & Capstick, C. (2004). Promising treatments for women with comorbid PTSD and substance use disorders. *American Journal of Psychiatry, 161,* 1426–1432.

Lehman, W. E. K., Greener, J. M., & Simpson, D. D. (2002). Assessing organizational readiness for change. *Journal of Substance Abuse Treatment, 22*(4), 197–209.

Marlatt, G. A., & Gordon, J. R. (1985). Relapse prevention. New York: Guilford.

McCarty, D., Gustafson, D. H., Wisdom, J. P., Ford, J., Dongseok, C., Molfenter, T., Capoccia, V., & Cotter, F. (2007). The Network for the Improvement of Addiction Treatment (NIATx): Enhancing access and retention. *Drug and Alcohol Dependence, 88,* 138–145.

McEvoy, P. M., & Nathan, P. (2007). Effectiveness of cognitive behavioral therapy for diagnostically heterogeneous groups: A benchmarking study. *Journal of Consulting and Clinical Psychology, 75*(2), 344–350.

McGovern, M. P., Alterman, A. I., Drake, K. M., & Dauten, A. P. (2008). Co-occurring PTSD and substance use disorders in addiction treatment settings. In K. T. Mueser and S. Rosenberg (Eds.), *Treating posttraumatic stress disorders in special populations*. Washington, DC: American Psychological Association Press.

McGovern, M. P., Clark, R. E., & Samnaliev, M. (2007). Medicaid beneficiaries with co-occurring substance use and psychiatric disorders: A multi-state application of the quadrant model. *Psychiatric Services, 58*(7), 949–954.

McGovern, M. P., Matzkin, A., & Giard, J. (2007). Assessing the dual diagnosis capability of addiction treatment services: The Dual Diagnosis Capability in Addiction Treatment (DDCAT) Index. *Journal of Dual Diagnosis, 3*(2), 111–123.

McGovern, M. P., & McLellan, A. T. (2008). The status of addiction treatment research with co-occurring substance use and psychiatric disorders. *Journal of Substance Abuse Treatment, 34*(1), 1–2.

McGovern, M. P., Wrisley, B. R., & Drake, R. E. (2005). Special section on relapse prevention: Relapse of substance use disorder and its prevention among persons with co-occurring disorders. *Psychiatric Services, 56,* 1270–1273.

McLellan, A. T., Lewis, D. C., O'Brien, C. P., & Kleber, H. D. (2000). Drug dependence, a chronic medical illness: Implications for treatment, insurance, and outcomes evaluation. *Journal of the American Medical Association, 284*(13), 1689–1695.

Najavits, L. M. (In press). Seeking safety: A new psychotherapy for posttraumatic stress disorder and substance use disorder. In P. Ouimette & P. Brown (Eds.), *Trauma and substance abuse: Causes, consequences, and treatment of comorbid disorders*. Washington, DC: American Psychological Association Press.

Randall, C. L., Thomas, S. E., & Thevos, A. K. (2001). Concurrent alcoholism and social anxiety disorder: A first step toward developing effective treatments. *Alcoholism: Clinical and Experimental Research, 25*(2), 210–220.

Substance Abuse and Mental Health Services Administration. (2002). *Report to Congress on the prevention and treatment of co-occurring substance abuse disorders and mental disorders*. Rockville, MD: Substance Abuse and Mental Health Services Administration, U.S. Department of Health and Human Services.

Weiss, R. D., Griffin, M. L., Kolodziej, M. E., Greenfield, S. F., Najavits, L. M., Daley, D. C., Doreau, H. R., & Hennen, J. A. (2007). A randomized trial of integrated group therapy versus group drug counseling for patients with bipolar disorder and substance dependence. *American Journal of Psychiatry, 164,* 100–107.

Recommended Reading

Co-occurring Disorders—General

Baker, A., & Velleman, R. (Eds.) (2007). *Clinical handbook of co-existing mental health and drug and alcohol problems.* New York: Routledge.

Brady, K. T., Halligan, P., & Malcolm, R. (1999). Dual diagnosis. In M. Galanter & H. D. Kleber (Eds.), *Textbook of substance abuse treatment* (pp. 475–484). Washington, DC: American Psychiatric Press.

Center for Substance Abuse Treatment. (1994, 1995). *Assessment and treatment of patients with co-existing mental illness and alcohol and other drug abuse.* Treatment Improvement Protocol (TIP) Series 9. (DHHS Publication No. [SMA] 95–306). Rockville, MD: Center for Substance Abuse Treatment, U.S. Department of Health and Human Services.

Center for Substance Abuse Treatment. (2005). *Substance abuse treatment for persons with co-occurring disorders.* Treatment Improvement Protocol (TIP) Series 42. (DHHS Publication No. [SMA] 05–3992). Rockville, MD: Substance Abuse and Mental Health Services Administration, U.S. Department of Health and Human Services.

Centre for Addiction and Mental Health. (2002). *Best practices: Concurrent mental health and substance use disorders.* Ottawa, Canada: Health Canada.

McGovern, M. P., Xie, H., Segal, S. R., Siembab, L., & Drake, R. E. (2006). Addiction treatment services and co-occurring disorders: Prevalence estimates, treatment practices, and barriers. *Journal of Substance Abuse Treatment, 31*(3), 267–275.

Mueser, K. T., Noordsy, D. L., Drake, R. E., & Fox, L. (2003). *Integrated treatment for dual disorders.* New York: The Guilford Press.

Substance Abuse and Mental Health Services Administration. (2002). *Report to Congress on the prevention and treatment of co-occurring substance abuse disorders and mental disorders.* Rockville, MD: Substance Abuse and Mental Health Services Administration, U.S. Department of Health and Human Services.

Substance Use Disorders—General

Margolis, R. D., & Zweben, J. E. (1998). *Treating patients with alcohol and other drug problems: An integrated approach.* Washington, DC: American Psychological Association.

McGovern, M. P., & Carroll, K. M. (2003). Evidence-based practices for substance use disorders. *Psychiatric Clinics of North America, 26*(4), 991–1010.

Miller, W. R., & Rollnick, S. (2002). *Motivational interviewing: Preparing people for change* (2nd ed.). New York: The Guilford Press.

Co-occurring Disorders—Anxiety and Substance Use Disorders

Barlow, D. H. (2002). *Anxiety and its disorders: The nature and treatment of anxiety and panic* (2nd ed.). New York: The Guilford Press.

CBT for Anxiety Disorders

Boston University. *David H. Barlow, Ph.D., A.B.P.P.: Treatment manuals.* Retrieved January 2008, from www.bu.edu/anxiety/dhb/treatmentmanuals.shtml.

Kushner, M. G., Abrams, K., & Borchardt, C. (2000). The relationship between anxiety disorders and alcohol use disorders: A review of major perspectives and findings. *Clinical Psychology Review, 20*(2), 149–171.

Randall, C. L., Thomas, S., & Thevos, A. K. (2001). Concurrent alcoholism and social anxiety disorder: A first step toward developing effective treatments. *Alcoholism: Clinical and Experimental Research, 25*(2), 210–220.

Co-occurring Disorders—Depression and Substance Use Disorders

Beck, A. T. , Rush, A. J., Shaw, B. F., & Emery, G. (1979). *Cognitive therapy of depression.* New York: The Guilford Press.

Burns, D. D. (1990, 1999). *The feeling good handbook.* New York: Penguin Books.

Brown, R. A., & Ramsey, S. E. (2000). Addressing comorbid depressive symptomatology in alcohol treatment. *Professional Psychology: Research and Practice, 31*(4), 418–422.

International Society for Interpersonal Psychotherapy. *Interpersonal therapy for depression therapy manual.* www.interpersonalpsychotherapy.org/index.html.

Co-occurring Disorders—Post-traumatic Stress and Substance Use Disorders

Najavits, L. M. (2001). *Seeking safety: A treatment manual for PTSD and substance abuse.* New York: The Guilford Press.

Ouimette, P., & Brown, P. J. (Eds.). (2002). *Trauma and substance abuse: Causes, consequences, and the treatment of comorbid disorders.* Washington, DC: American Psychological Association.

Seeking safety: A model for trauma/PTSD and substance abuse. www.seekingsafety.org

Co-occurring Disorders—Personality and Substance Use Disorders

Evans, K., & Sullivan, J. M. (1990). *Dual diagnosis.* New York: The Guilford Press.

Evans, K., & Sullivan, J. M. (1990). *Step study counseling with the dual disordered client.* Center City, MN: Hazelden.

Linehan, M. M., Schmidt, H., III, Dimeff, L. A., Craft, J. C., Kanter, J., & Comtois, K. A. (1999). Dialectical behavior therapy for patients with borderline personality disorder and drug-dependence. *American Journal on Addictions 8*(4), 279–292.

Dialectical Behavior Therapy

University of Washington. *Marsha M. Linehan.* Retrieved January 2008, from http://faculty.washington.edu/linehan.

Co-occurring Disorders—Adolescents

Riggs, P. D. (2003). Treating adolescents for substance abuse and comorbid psychiatric disorders. *Science & Practice Perspectives, 2*(1), 18–32.

Co-occurring Disorders—Web-Based Bibliography

Treatment Improvement Exchange. *Dual disorders special topic.* Retrieved January 2008, from http://www.treatment.org/Topics/dual_documents.html.

•   •   •